The
Decision

By Juan Gomez Jr.

THE DECISION

Dedication

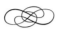

First and foremost, I would like to thank God for his many blessings. I dedicate this to all of you in my life that are the true definition of family. Especially to my children Jazmyn, Gabriel, Ethan, my mother Sally, my sister Pamela and her wonderful family, and to my brothers Jorge and Anthony. Without your love and support none of this would be possible. Thank you all for always being there. I love you all. To all those in hospitals, and treatment centers around the world fighting illnesses with the ultimate weapons, your faith that the lord will provide, hope that everything will be okay and especially the love in your hearts. With everything that goes on in your life, you all never stop fighting. You all are the true inspirations and to that I want to say thank you.

Table of Contents

Chapter 1

"And I pray for Aunt Yolanda, Aunt Ruthie, Jazmyn, Gabriel, and Daddy. Please watch over us and please heal Jazzy, Bubby, and me. Let us not feel pain anymore. Please take the cancers away from us and don't let us feel sickie anymore so Jazzy, Bubby, and me can play outside and not go to the hospital. Thank you, Lord, for everything you have done for us. In Jesus name we pray, Amen."

"Very good, Annabelle. Thank you for that lovely prayer," Michael says. "Okay, my little soldiers, are you ready for body check?"

"Ready!" scream the kids.

"Head?"

"Check!"

"Tummy?"

"Check!"

"Boogies?"

"Daddy!" the kids shout as Michael laughs.

"I was just seeing if you guys were paying attention. Okay, princess, you're first. Let's get you tucked in. How's my little bubble?"

"Awesome!"

"That's my little princess, here is your goodnight bear. There, you are all set now to go have sweet dreams. I love you. Goodnight!"

As she snuggles with her bear, she says, "Night night, Daddy. Love you."

Michael shuts the door.

"Okay, Gabriel, you're up, buddy! How is your stomach?"

"It hurts a little."

"I know buddy, but your medicine should be working to help you fight those meanies. Do you want me to hang around?"

"No, it's okay. I'm getting sleepy now."

"Okay buddy, you rest up."

"Wait!"

"What is it?"

"Monster check!"

"You're right, buddy. I'm sorry. Nope, not in the closet. Nope, not under the bed. Looks like you're good to sleep."

"Thank you, Daddy. I love you."

Michael smiles back at him. "I love you too, buddy. Goodnight."

"Goodnight, Daddy."

Michael closes the door halfway. "Okay, Annabelle, you're up. You know the drill."

"Yeah, yeah, I'm okay."

"You know I must check sweetie. Do you want a monster check?"

"Daddy, I'm 12," she says with a look.

"Okay, I'm sorry, but you know you will always be my little girl no matter how old you are. Goodnight, I love you."

"I love you too. Goodnight!"

Michael closes the door and makes his way to his aunt. "Aunt Ruthie, how are you feeling?"

"Tired. I'm drained."

"How is your sugar level?"

"It's good. I just checked it."

"Okay, well let me know if you need anything."

"I will, Michael. I know I'm ready for this bed," she says, getting comfortable.

"I love you, Aunt Ruthie. Goodnight!"

"Goodnight, Michael. I love you too."

Michael shuts off the lights and closes the door. "Goodnight everyone! I love you all! Gabriel, Annabelle put down those electronics. It's time for bed!"

"Aw man!" the kids say as Michael laughs to himself.

"What am I going to do with you guys? Whew, what a day. Lord thank you for letting everyone have a good day today and for letting them make it through another."

Michael walks out to the living room to find his sister straightening up. "Yolanda, what are you doing?"

"Cleaning—what does it look like I'm doing?"

"You don't have to do that. I will take care of it."

"It's okay. I will clean out here. You get the kitchen."

"Okay, sis, I'm on it."

As Michael walks into the kitchen, he turns to Yolanda. "I'll tell you this—I love them, but it looks like a hurricane came through here."

They both share a laugh.

"You got that right!" Yolanda says, "With all the toys they have and rooms to put them in, how they end up out here is beside me."

"I wouldn't change a thing about them. Well, except to take their illnesses away."

"I know, Michael. I know you would if you could, but you have to trust and have faith in God."

"I do, Yolanda, but it's not fair. It's not fair that Jazmyn, my princess, has neuroblastoma and is only 3! Next there is my little buddy, Gabriel, with what they think is DSRCT, and he is 10. Finally, there is Annabelle diagnosed with progeria, and she is 12! I mean...why? Why would such a loving god do that?"

"I understand your frustration, but it's not for us to understand why. You must just be there for them. Keep showing them what you have been teaching all of us—to have hope, faith, and love. That's all you can do right now."

"I know, Yolanda. I just wish there was a way to help them. I know God has a plan; I just wish he would let me peek at it. Do you understand?"

"I do, Michael, but you're not alone. We are here for you and the kids."

"I know that, sis. I appreciate all that you and Aunt Ruthie do for us."

"We are family, Michael. That is what family does for each other—to always be there through good and bad times. We always stick together."

"Thank you, Yolanda, but you know who I wish were here?"

"Anna?"

"Yes. I miss her so much. I miss her laughter and the way she smiled with those beautiful blue eyes of hers. I especially miss the way she commanded attention when she walked into a room."

"Don't forget, man, she could sing!"

"That too. It was as if she had a voice of an angel! Speaking of angels, I know she is up there in heaven showing them all up with her singing and dancing."

They laugh.

"Yes, she is, but she is home, Michael. That is what one thing you must take comfort in."

"I do… it's just that she is—well, was—the love of my life."

"You fell for that girl the minute she smiled at you."

"That I did. To be honest with you, when I first saw her, it was as if I knew her already. Like I had dreamt her to life, because when she smiled at me it was over."

"She knew what she was doing. She told me that the minute she saw you, she knew you were the one."

"How does that work? All we did was stare at each other, then she smiled, and…I don't know. It was as if my life depended on me going over to talk to her. You know?"

"Oh yes, I know what you're talking about. But she did say she knew you were the reason she was there. As a matter of fact, she didn't want to go out that night, but her friends made her get out of the house."

"Really?"

"Yes, she said that as she sat there wanting to go home, you walked in, and she knew at that moment why she was there."

Michael laughs playfully. "That's right!"

"Shut up! Don't get big-headed."

"I'm just playing around. But seriously, I only walked in there to use the restroom."

"You did?"

"I walked in, saw her, and, honestly Yolanda, only one light was shining bright and it was on her."

Yolanda laughs. "You never really stood a chance!"

"You've got that right! I just can't explain it. I walked in, saw her, we locked eyes, she smiled, then I went to her. I'd even forgotten the reason why I walked in there!" Michael and Yolanda both laugh. "In all seriousness, you know how they say that the world disappears when you're with the one?"

"I know the feeling"

"It wasn't like that. I looked into those beautiful blue eyes of hers, and it was as if we were in another world. I didn't hear any noise, it felt like nothing was around us. It was just her and me sitting there. I'm trying to describe it the best way I can, but it's the type of feeling you can't put into words. Do you understand what I'm trying to say?"

"You have no idea. It's funny you say that, because she said the same exact thing."

"She did?"

"Yes, she said that when you finally came and sat down, nothing else mattered at that moment—like this world didn't exist. She said it was then she knew in her heart you were the one she had been waiting for."

"She said that? I had no idea."

"You men never do." They both laugh. "You know, she told me the first words you both said to each other. Do you remember them?"

"Of course I do! But hey, I had no control over that. It was as if my brain had gone into overdrive and was speaking for me. The only words I could say were, 'Where have you been?' I have no idea why I said that."

"Yes, but her response was what?"

"Waiting for you," they both say together.

"I was struck by that," Michael says. "We were married soon after. Then we had three beautiful children… and then she was taken from us."

"Michael she wasn't taken. God created you both for each other. The time you had with her was a blessing from above."

"I know it was, but it still hurts not having her here. It's not for me to argue or blame God for the reasons he wanted her home. I just don't understand why that at the very moment she was on her way home that guy thought he could drive home drunk—it's beyond me."

"I know it hurts, Michael, but she is alive in those kids and in you. Just try to understand that."

"Thank you, and I do understand that. It's just I wish she were here."

"I know you do, but we are here, and whatever you need from us we are here for you all."

"That means a lot."

"Well it's getting late. I better take myself to bed."

"Okay, Yolanda, and thanks again for the talk."

"Anytime. Like I said, we are here whenever you need us."

"Do you need me to tuck you in?"

"If you don't get out of here with that!" They both laugh.

"Okay, sis, goodnight. I love you."

"I love you too, Michael. Goodnight."

"Wow, it is getting late. Where does the time fly? I better get myself to bed as well."

As Michael prepares for bed, he does what he always does: he prays.

"Lord, thank you for all you have done for us and thank you for all your blessings. Please heal my children from their illnesses. Lord, please heal my aunt Ruthie from her diabetes. Please watch over us as I know in my heart you always do. Give me the strength every day to handle my responsibilities. Give me strength, Lord, to carry on every day, and in turn, give strength to my children, as they are yours. Please watch over this world, Lord,, as we are in such turmoil. Guide us to safety, and arm us with your knowledge to care for one another as you do.

"I know you have a plan for all of us, Lord, but please let me know what I must do to heal and save my children from their suffering. I will do whatever is asked of me, Lord, just please tell me. I have the utmost faith and trust in you, Lord, and forgive me, but it's just so hard to see not only my children but many around this world going through these illnesses and the problems that come from them. Please give us all the strength to carry on. Help them all, Lord, to defeat whatever is trying to attack your children.

"In your heavenly name, I pray, Lord. Amen."

Chapter 2

"What you are doing?"

"Hi princess. Of course you would be the first one up. Give me those little cheeks."

Jazmyn giggles.

"How is your bubble?"

"It's okay, Daddy, my bubble is still here, see!"

"Don't touch it, princess. What do you want to watch?"

"Cartoons!" she says with excitement.

"Okay, princess, let me finish cooking breakfast, and I will turn on the television, okay?"

"'Kay!"

As Michael prepares breakfast, he sees Jazmyn growing impatient.

"Princess, where is the remote?"

"Here Daddy!"

"Thank you. Okay, here are your cartoons. Go ahead and watch your shows while Daddy finishes up breakfast."

"'Kay!"

God, I love her so much. Okay, time to finish before everyone comes out. They should be out here any minute.

As Michael finishes up breakfast, he hears running coming towards him.

"Daddy!" scream the other children.

"Good morning, soldiers. How are we today?"

"Good!" they both say loudly.

"I am glad to hear that. Did you both brush your teeth? Gabriel, I'm looking at you, buddy."

"Aw, man!" he says as he walks away.

"Annabelle, what about you sweetie?"

"Yup! See!"

"I see, sweetie. How are you feeling?"

"Okay, daddy, but my chest feels a little weird."

"What? What do you mean it feels weird?"

"It just feels like someone is squeezing it."

"Do we need to go to the hospital? I mean, adventure land?"

"No, I will be okay. It doesn't hurt. It just feels like it's being squeezed."

"I think we should go anyways to be safe—just to make sure nothing is going on."

"No, it's okay! If it hurts, I will let you know."

"Okay, Annabelle. Only you know your body, so I am trusting you. If at any point you don't feel like you're okay, just let me know right away. Go ahead and watch television with your sister. When Gabriel comes back, breakfast should be done."

"Okay. Hey, Daddy, what is the password to the tablet?"

"Nice try, sweetie."

"Hey, it was worth a shot!"

"I will give you that. Like I always say, you never know something until you try. That's like life—if you don't go for what you want, you've already failed. Remember that, okay?"

"Yes, Daddy, I hear you."

"Okay, sweetie, I logged you on. Go ahead and do whatever it is you do on that thing."

"Way ahead of you!"

"Wait! Where is my cheek?"

"Ahh, right here!"

"Okay, sweetie, you can now continue. Love you."

"Love you too!"

Gabriel comes running in.

"About time, buddy! What were you doing for so long?"

"All clean. See!" He shows off his teeth.

"That's good, buddy. I don't want stinky breath, and you know girls don't like that either."

"Dad!"

Michael laughs. "You will understand one day. Go ahead and watch television with your sisters."

"Okay!"

"Wait! I need a cheek."

"Here it is!"

"Okay, buddy, go ahead. Breakfast is almost done."

"Good. I'm hungry!"

"I know you are. Don't worry, it's almost done. Daddy is just late getting it out. I wonder where Yolanda and Aunt Ruthie are?" He then shouts out to them: "Hey, sis! Aunt Ruthie! Oh, I hear someone coming."

"Good morning, Michael. Hey cuties."

"Good morning, Aunt Yolanda!" says the children.

"Good morning, Yolanda. How are you today?"

"I am good. I just couldn't decide what to wear. Honestly, I think my brain shuts down on me sometimes. I can't even think of simple tasks like what to wear or what shoes to go with it."

"You are showing your age, sis." They share a laugh.

"Hey, you're the one with the gray hairs on your head."

"That's the style that's in now. Right, soldiers?"

"Nope!" they say jokingly.

"Whatever! I know I look good, but if you want me to pick out your clothes, Yolanda, I can."

She smirks. "I think I am good in that department. Besides you seem to not have any fashion sense."

"What are you talking about? I should be on a fashion cover or something."

Everyone laughs.

"Look Michael, sport shirts and jerseys are not fashion."

"Say what you want about fashion, but sports are always in style. It makes a statement."

"What, that you are advertising for them?"

"I am representing the home team. You're just jealous."

"I love you, but we need to take you to the store and buy you some fashion sense."

"Okay, what do you see me in then?"

"I don't know—maybe polo shirts or button-downs. You know... something with style."

"I have style!"

"We live in Tampa, and all you wear are either baseball, football, or hockey shirts or jerseys. I'm sorry, but that is not style."

"You're crazy. You don't know what you're talking about."

"You're 38 years old and dress like a frat boy. I mean...your poor kids. They inherited your sports look. Just look at them with their Tampa Bay pajamas. Who are you trying to fool? You are training them!"

Michael laughs. "They look good though!"

"You know, if Anna were here, this frat boy look you have going on wouldn't fly. Oh, I'm sorry, Michael. I didn't mean to bring her up."

"No, it's okay. You are right; she wouldn't have let me leave the room with what I have on. She would have made me go back and change."

"That she would have done."

"I tell you what, I will make you a deal. After we take Aunt Ruthie to her doctor's appointment or—even better because today is going to be a long one for her—while she is there, we will go shopping. Sound good?"

"It's about time!"

"Okay, Yolanda. Whatever puts a smile on your face."

"Sounds good to me, but if you tell me to give you a cheek right now, I am going to slap you."

They both laugh.

"What? Just one cheek?"

"If you don't go somewhere with that, I tell you what. Anyway, breakfast smells good. Anna trained you very well."

Michael smiles. "Yes, she did. She was training me the minute I said, 'Hi, my name is Michael.'"

Yolanda smiles. "Yeah, she was."

"Okay, soldiers, come and get it!"

"Yay!" the kids yell excitedly.

"I haven't seen Aunt Ruthie yet. I wonder where she could be?"

"I think she is in the bathroom still. I don't think feels too good today."

"Is she okay?"

"I think so, but let me go check on her."

"Okay, Yolanda. Thank you. Princess, let's get in your chair."

"Up, Daddy!" she says with her arms in the air.

"Okay, princess, there you are. Let me lock in you tight, and there—you're all set. Before we say grace, do you guys want juice or milk?"

"Juice!"

"Okay, buddy. Annabelle, what would you like?"

"Milk for me, please."

"Princess, what about you?"

"Juice."

"Okay, soldiers! Coming right up!"

In comes Yolanda. "Hey, Michael, look who I found!"

"Hey Aunt Ruthie, good morning. Yolanda told me you weren't feeling too well, and you were in the bathroom. Is everything okay?"

"Good morning, Michael. Hi, babies."

"Good morning, Aunt Ruthie!" the kids say with smiles.

"You and Yolanda worry too much. I am fine."

"Yes, but we care about you."

"I am okay now. I woke up not feeling so hot, but I am good now."

"Okay, Aunt Ruthie. It's nice to see that beautiful face of yours. Give me a cheek."

She smiles. "You are something else. Bring it in."

He plants a big kiss on her. "That's all I wanted. I have your breakfast ready for you."

"What flavor is on the menu today?"

"Your favorite: vanilla!"

"You know how to spoil me, don't you?"

They all share a laugh.

"Okay, it looks like everyone has their drinks and food. Let's say grace."

"If you don't mind, Michael, I would like to say it today."

"Okay, Aunt Ruthie."

"Lord, we are thankful for this delicious meal we are about to eat and thankful for these babies being here as well as Michael and Yolanda. We give you all the thanks in all the blessings you give us and in everything you allow us to do in Jesus' name. Amen."

"Thank you for that, Aunt Ruthie. Okay everyone, let's eat."

As Michael sat there looking around the table, he couldn't help but thank God for blessing him with such a family.

"You know everyone, this right here is family."

"What do you mean, Daddy?" says Annabelle, confused.

"I will tell you all something: remember these moments. Remember all those that are in your life and be thankful for moments like these. For there is an old saying—a family that eats and prays together, stays together."

"Like we do, Daddy?"

"That's right, buddy, because no matter what always make time for your family. Everyone understand that?"

"We understand, Daddy," say the children.

"Aunt Ruthie, Yolanda, that goes for you two, as well."

"We hear you, Michael."

"Okay, just checking. Speaking of time, let's get finished, then dressed. We must go soon. Aunt Ruthie, when we take you to your appointment, are okay with us going to do a little shopping?"

"Yes, I am okay with that. Besides, today is going to be a long one. They seem to want to check for everything."

"I just wanted to make sure. I don't feel right just dropping you off like that."

"Michael, it's fine. I don't like you all to wait around for me anyways."

"No, it's no problem. We don't mind it at all."

"You have a 12-, 10-, and 3-year-old. I hardly think they like waiting. Besides, they see enough doctors and hospitals. Just go ahead and do whatever it is you guys want to do."

"Okay, Aunt Ruthie, thank you."

"Just out of curiosity, what are you guys going shopping for?"

Yolanda smiles. "He is finally going to dress like an adult."

"What?!"

"Yeah, Daddy, no more sport clothes," says Annabelle, laughing.

"And I can get shoes, right Daddy?"

"Yes, buddy, all of us are going shopping."

"Well, do me one favor, Michael."

"Anything, Aunt Ruthie. What do you need?"

"For you to retire that look of yours!"

Everyone shares a laugh.

"Hey! But you're right; it's time I guess. Yolanda and I had a long talk about it."

"Well, good. I didn't want to be the one that brought it up, but since everyone agrees, right babies?"

"That's right, Daddy!" yell the children, laughing as Yolanda joins in.

"I told you, Michael."

"Okay, okay, you all win. Is everyone done?"

"I am, Daddy!"

"That's good, buddy. Please go get dressed."

"Okay!" he shouts as he runs off.

"Annabelle, go ahead and get dressed as well, please."

"Okay," she says, leaving.

"Princess, let's get you cleaned up and smelling and looking like a princess."

"'Kay," she says, giggling.

"I will be back. Do you two need more time?"

"We are fine, Michael. Go get those beautiful children of yours ready."

"Okay, Yolanda. Hey, should I go change?"

"No!" they both shout.

"Wow, that was a quick response."

Yolanda and Aunt Ruthie laugh. "No, it's best the salesperson sees you the way you are. That way they know what they are working with."

"Okay, ha-ha, I see your point. Just wait I am going to laugh when both of you lose your fashion sense."

"Michael, you are going to be waiting a long time on that one," says Yolanda, laughing.

"Go ahead. Laugh it up you two. We shall see. Okay, princess, let's go get you ready. Yolanda, do you mind cleaning this up for me? I'm sorry to ask."

"Michael, it's no problem. Go get them dressed. I will take care of it."

"Thank you, sis. You're the best."

As Yolanda cleans, Michael gets Jazmyn ready.

"Okay, soldiers, everyone ready, set to go?"

"I am, Daddy."

"I know, princess. That's because I got you ready remember? Now, your bubby and sissy… that is a different story. Soldiers!" he shouts out.

"Coming!"

"Okay buddy. Annabelle we are waiting on you!"

"I'm here! You can't rush pretty, Daddy!"

"You're right, sweetie, but you know you are already pretty when you wake up."

"Thank you, Daddy."

"Anytime, sweetie. Okay, buddy, where are you? I thought you said you were coming!"

"Right here. I couldn't find my shoe."

"Let me guess, that is why you need new ones, right?"

"Right!"

"Okay, soldiers, now that we are all here let's hop in the car and take Aunt Ruthie to her magic land."

"Adventure land, Daddy?"

"No buddy. We are taking her to another magic land that's just for her."

"Oh, okay."

"Yolanda, Aunt Ruthie, are you ready?"

"I am. What about you Aunt Ruthie?"

"Yes, I guess. Let's get this over with."

"Okay everyone, let's go."

They all pile into the car and head off.

"Now, Aunt Ruthie, please tell Doctor Johnson everything that has been going on with you. Like your blood pressure and especially how when you woke up you weren't feeling too good."

"Yes, Michael, I know. It's sweet you worry about me, but I will be fine."

"I'm just saying. Doctors don't know what really is going on unless you speak up. You hear me back there, soldiers?"

"Yes, Daddy, we hear you."

"Just making sure everyone heard me. I'm serious about what I said, Aunt Ruthie. Please don't leave anything out."

"Yes, Michael."

"Thank you. I know I'm what you might call a cautious person, but I care about all your well beings."

"I know you do, Michael, but just continue to have faith and let God guide you."

"I will and always do."

They arrive at the doctor's office."

"Daddy this is not adventure land!"

"I know sweetie, but as I said before, this magic land is just for Aunt Ruthie."

"So she can get better, Daddy?"

"Yes, buddy. Just like you three have your potions to make you guys feel better, Aunt Ruthie has hers here."

"Oh, okay."

"Let's go in, soldiers."

"No, Michael, you can just drop me off here. There is no need for all of you guys to come in."

"No, it's okay. Besides I want to say hi to Teresa."

"Don't lie to me. You just want to make sure she has me down for a full work-up."

Michael smiles. "No, I just want to make sure you're going to be okay. Also, I really do want to say hi to Teresa. Besides like I said before, I don't want to drop you off and leave. Okay, soldiers, let's all go in for a minute, and then we can go shopping."

"Okay," say the children, jumping out of the car.

"Ladies first. Remember this buddy: in order to be a gentleman, you must act like one. For example, it's always ladies first and hold the door open."

Gabriel holds the door with Michael. "Like this, Daddy?"

"That's right, buddy, good job!"

They all walk into the office.

"Hi, Teresa. How are you today?"

"Oh, hi guys. I am having a wonderful day today. Thank you for asking. How is everyone doing?"

"Well, we are as good as we are going to be."

"I understand. It's like they say, if you woke up, then that is a blessing."

"Amen to that."

"Ruth, Dr. Johnson will be ready for you in a bit, okay?"

"Yes, dear, thank you."

"Aunt Ruthie, we don't mind waiting with you."

"Michael, if I have to tell you one more time that I will be okay, then we are going to have problems."

"Yes ma'am. I hear you loud and clear."

"Please do me that favor I asked and dress like the person I know you are."

"Yes, Aunt Ruthie, I will. Okay, soldiers, say goodbye to Aunt Ruthie and Miss Teresa.

"Goodbye Aunt Ruthie. Goodbye Miss Teresa," say the children as they walk out.

"Bye, cuties. You have such well-mannered children, Michael."

"Thank you for that, but I can't take all the credit. Aunt Ruthie, if you happen to get out early or need anything, give me a call."

"Goodbye Michael."

"Okay, Aunt Ruthie, I love you."

"I love you too."

"I will be back soon, Teresa. If she needs anything, don't hesitate to call."

"Okay, Michael. Will do. Bye," she says smiling.

"Daddy, why did you say I love you even though we are coming back?"

"Well, Annabelle, sweetie, you never know what God has planned for us next, so whenever you say goodnight, goodbye, or something of that nature, you always say 'I love you' to ones that you feel that way towards. You must always take every opportunity you have to tell them how you feel before you leave."

"Like you do, Daddy?"

"Exactly, buddy. As I say that to you all before I leave you. God forbid it but if he has his plan in place, I want you all to know how much I love you."

"You mean like die, Daddy?"

"Unfortunately, sweetie, sometimes God's plan is for us to go back home with him, but yes, in that sense always make sure your loved ones know that you love them. Never let an opportunity go by. If you have a chance to say how you feel, then say it. Everyone understand?"

"We love you, Daddy," say the children smiling.

"I love you all, too. Okay, soldiers, what say we go ahead and get going and go find Daddy some style?"

"And shoes, too! Right, Daddy?"

"Yes buddy. Everyone will get to pick out something at the store."

"Yay!" the children say with excitement.

"It's about time, Michael."

"Yolanda, I already agreed to go, so let's go ahead and get this over with. Where do you want to go?"

"To go fix you up the way Anna did."

"Hey!"

"Calm down, I'm just playing around. But seriously let's go to Today's Fashion. They should have something for you to dress like an adult."

"Yeah, Daddy, plus they have cute shoes there!"

"Okay, Annabelle, it sounds like a winner."

Yolanda leans over to the children. "You guys ready for Daddy to dress his age?"

"You're old, Daddy!" say the children playfully.

"Lord, what am I going to do with you guys?"

Chapter 3

"Okay, everyone, we are finally here. Soldiers, how are we feeling? Is everyone good to go in?"

"Yeah," say the children as they hop out of the car.

"Well, cheer up, soldiers! Where are those beautiful smiles at? Do I need to get those cheeks?"

"No, we are fine, Daddy!"

"Okay, that's it. Let me get those cheeks. Come here."

"Daddy, that is only for when we are at home," says Annabelle, walking away.

"Yeah, Daddy," said Gabriel, chiming in.

"Well fine. I will just get them at home then."

"I hate to be the one to tell you this Michael, but it looks like they are growing up on you."

"I know right! It feels like it was just yesterday I was wiping their butts. Now it's electronics-this and download-that. I am telling you, Yolanda, I am going to blink, and they are going to graduate."

"No offense, Michael, but with the way you keep treating them, I would play it by ear."

"What? Why would you say something like that?"

"No, I didn't mean it like that, but look at them. Yes, they are sick, but you keep reminding them about it all the time. You don't exactly give them the confidence to succeed."

"With what they are going through I constantly worry about them."

"I understand that, and you should, but don't remind them all the time that they are sick by asking if they are okay every minute. They don't need you to remind them of it. Forgive me if I am out of place with this, but they talk to me all the time on how much you worry and stress about them every minute of the day. It stresses them out. They feel like it's as if you don't think they are going to make it."

"Yolanda, look. It is my job to make sure they are okay every day, and yes, I may go overboard sometimes, but I love them so much."

"That is understandable, but don't make them feel a certain type of way that makes them think they can't dream."

"It's like this, Yolanda. I have the ultimate faith in the Lord and in my children to make it. As a matter of fact, everyone please gather around me. I am sorry if I treat you guys differently, but I care about you all so much. If you have dreams, go for it. Never—and I repeat—never let anyone, including myself, take that from you. You all—and, yes, Yolanda, I am talking to you too—have something nobody can take from you: the love of God. That is the most powerful weapon in this world. It is the type of love that many on this earth search for their entire lives but fail to realize that it was gifted to us the minute we were born. He loves us all so much. He believes in us so much to succeed in life. It's the same way I believe in you all. Yes, you three have these meanies trying to get you, but you're stronger than anything that is trying. Never lose hope. Never lose your faith in God and in yourselves. Never lose the love you have for Him and never give up on your dreams. Is everyone clear on that?"

"Yes, I am sorry."

"Me too, Daddy."

"No, my loves, I am the one who is sorry for making you feel that way in the first place. I am sorry for putting you through what is already a difficult journey that you all are going through. Come here, soldiers, let me hug you guys." Michael goes to hug each one. "Seriously, did you all understand what I said?"

"We did, Daddy!" the children say cheerfully.

"Yolanda?"

"I understand, Michael."

"Okay. With all that said, what say we do what we came for and shop?"

"Yay!" they say with excitement.

"Let's go in."

"Ladies first, right, Daddy?"

"That's right, buddy. I am proud of you."

As they walk in, they are greeted by a cheerful employee. "Hi, welcome to Today's Fashion. Is there anything I can help you with?"

"Yes, please point us in the direction to fix my brother's style and find him some fashion."

"Hey! Michael says swiftly as the employee smiles.

"Yes, the men's section is on the right towards the back. You should be able to find something suitable for him there."

"Okay, thank you."

"Sure, and if you need any help, we will be more than happy to assist you."

"Thank you. Okay everyone, we know what we came for. Let's get to it."

"Yes, Lord, thank you!" Yolanda says sarcastically.

"Let's see, what we do have here? Oh, sis, what about this? It's colorful."

"Michael, if you don't put that down and find real clothes, then there is going to be an issue!"

"Yeah, Daddy!"

"What? Sweetie, you don't like it?"

"No!"

"Wow! Even my 12-year-old has more fashion sense than I do. Okay, Miss Fashionista, what look should I go with then?"

"You should look like DJ El Mas Sin Cero."

"What? Who?"

"Daddy! Pick up your phone and use it occasionally. He's not only the hottest DJ but he also knows how to dress."

"That's it. I am cancelling the internet!"

Annabelle laughs. "Daddy, you can't cancel the internet."

Yolanda begins to laugh as well.

"What, Tuggy? Do you have something you want to say?"

"Hey, I hate that name!"

"Well then, how about you three ladies go over to your sections, and my buddy and I will look over here. Right, Gabriel?"

"Yup!"

"Look, buddy, they have so much Tampa fan gear here…"

"No!" Yolanda and Annabelle yell.

"Wow! The way both of you said that, it was as if you two rehearsed it."

"Michael, absolutely no fan gear! Find men's clothes! That is the reason we are here. Just think to yourself, 'What Anna would buy?'"

"Yeah, yeah. I hear you. You ladies just go over to your sections. We have this handled. Hey buddy, check this out. This is nice. Are they gone?"

"Yup."

"Okay, buddy, don't judge me, but never be afraid to ask for help when you need to."

Michael sees an employee walking by. "Excuse me, miss."

"Hi!"

"I am sorry for asking, but what is your name?"

"My name is Jessica. What can I help you with today?"

"I am what you call someone that is fashion less."

Jessica smiles at him. "So, you're one of those guys, huh?"

"Yes. I am afraid so. It has been brought to my attention recently."

"Well, we have many styles to choose from. Let me ask you this, what are you most comfortable in?"

"That's the thing. I am comfortable with my fan gear."

"I see that."

"It works for me, but apparently not for others in my family."

Gabriel giggles.

"Yes, well, definitely follow me. Here we have button-downs, long-sleeve, short-sleeve, and polos. What do you see yourself in?"

"To be honest, I am clueless about all this fashion stuff. My—Well… let's just say someone used to style me."

"Oh, I'm sorry."

"No, it's okay. It's just that I am new at all of this again."

"I understand. If you don't mind me saying, she must have had good taste if she picked you."

"I wouldn't say that, but yes, admittingly she had better fashion sense than I did."

"Okay, well fashion is not just about the clothes."

"It's not?"

"I am not supposed to say this, but don't buy what is in style. Instead, buy what you feel. Fashion is a statement."

"I am sorry, but I am lost."

"For example, you wouldn't wear a suit to bed, right?"

"Well, of course not."

"Exactly. You would wear a suit to church, meetings, or anywhere you want to make a statement that you are successful. Don't get me wrong, I don't mean financially but in the general sense—as if you are telling someone 'I am important.' Why do you think someone in business wear suits?"

"To be honest I never understood that. I know that in church, it's your Sunday best."

"Well in business they are not saying, 'I have money.' They are making a statement that they someone you'd want to do business with. But appearances can be deceiving."

"What do you mean by that?"

"Say there are two people who walk into a bank. One is wearing a $1,000 suit, and the other has on jeans and a t-shirt. Who do you think the staff will approach first?"

"Well, the suit, of course."

"Exactly. But the person in the suit is there to get a loan. While the person in jeans and a t-shirt is there to deposit a large check. You see, fashion can be deceiving. That is why you never judge anyone by the way they look. Just like it says in the Bible. Matthew 7:1-2 says 'Judge not, that ye be not judged. For with what judgment ye judge, ye shall be judged: and with what measure ye mete, it shall be measured to you again.'"

"Amen to that."

"So, pick out what and how you feel that day. If you want to tell the world, 'I am comfortable,' then wear what you have on. But if you want to tell everyone, 'I am of age,' then I would find something more suitable to that nature. With what I gather from your style now, I would suggest polos and jeans."

"Really? I thought I would have to wear those slacks over there or something like it."

"No, actually, it's the new business casual. So, if you really want to dress your age, I would go with that look, but since you have this sporty look to you, I suggest golf shirts."

"Golf shirts?"

"Yes, I would definitely recommend that for you. They are sporty, comfortable, and made from great material. Like these over here. Like this blue one."

"Oh, okay. I think I have the general idea now. I will look around and take your suggestions into consideration. Thank you."

"My pleasure. And one final piece of advice: I would stick with light colors like that blue shirt you are holding. It brings out those hypnotizing eyes of yours."

Michael laughs bashfully. "Thank you again. I will take your advice on that."

"Any time. And if you need anything else, I won't be too far away."

"Okay, thank you." At that moment Michael notices Yolanda, Jazmyn, and Annabelle. "Oh, hi ladies. Did you three find anything you like?"

"You're an idiot, Michael."

"What?"

"She was clearly hitting on you."

"No, she wasn't."

"Oh, yes she was. 'Hypnotizing eyes,' 'I won't be too far away,' you really didn't notice that?"

"She was just being helpful. Besides, it is her job to help customers find the right clothes."

"Like I said. You're an idiot."

Michael laughs it off. "Anyways, I think I am going with her suggestions and taking these golf shirts. What do you think?"

"Go for it. I agree with her. They do look like a proper style for you."

"Daddy, I have to have these shoes!"

"Okay, sweetie, but did you find any clothes?"

"No, just these please."

"Okay, sweetie, whatever makes you smile."

"Yes!"

"What about Tuggy?"

"Michael!"

He laughs. "I am just messing with you. But seriously, did you find anything you liked?"

"Yes, I found a couple things."

"Princess, what about you?"

"I found her some really cute outfits and shoes."

"Pretty, Daddy!"

"I know you are, princess. Okay, buddy, looks like it's your turn. Let's go over here to the big boys' section."

As they make their way over, Gabriel runs to the shoes. "Daddy look! They have Pudgies!"

"What?"

"Pudgies!" he says with excitement.

"Yolanda, I am lost. What are those?"

"Seriously, Michael, get on the internet sometime."

"With what time? Okay, buddy, get your whatever-you-call-them."

"Yes!"

"Michael, in all seriousness, that employee was hitting on you."

"Okay, Yolanda. If you say so."

"As a matter of fact. When was the last time you dated?"

"You know I don't want to talk about that. Besides I don't need anyone. I have you guys. Right, princess?"

"Yup!"

"Well, I think you need an outlet. Go ask her out and have a night to yourself. It has been two years already. It is time for you to get out and be with someone other than us. You're with us 24 hours a day."

"Exactly. You are proving my point without me saying anything."

"No, I was letting you know to go out and get away from all this that is going on."

"Who will be there just in case something happens? That is my biggest fear."

"Michael, you can't be afraid 24 hours a day about things that might happen. I will give you an example. What if you go out and nothing happens? You are constantly on the move; you sleep, what, fours a night? If that? You need to go out at some point and, for once, have fun. Get your mind off all this worrying and self-doubt you have."

"I appreciate what you are trying to say, but I think I am okay for now."

"All I am trying to say to you is that it's not healthy for you not to move on. Yes, Anna was the love of your life, and maybe she was the one God intended for you to be with, but he called her back home for a reason."

"I know the reason; he was short an angel and wanted her back home with him in the kingdom of heaven."

"That is what I am trying to tell you. She is at home with our father, walking with Jesus and singing amongst the angels. She is happy. Probably not with what is going on here, but she is happy in the sense that she is with the Lord, and she knows all this is going on according to his plan. Do you think she would be happy with the way you are now? To see you like this?"

"You are probably right, Yolanda, but I have nothing to give anyone. When Anna was called back home, she took everything I had left. Do you understand?"

"Look at your kids. Look at how great a father you are to them; at how great a nephew you are with the way you treat Aunt Ruthie; and do not to forget how you are a wonderful brother to have."

"I appreciate that, Yolanda, but still, I feel that way in my heart."

"Your heart is still beating right?"

"Yes, it is."

"Look, the faith and love you have for God after everything that happened to you and what is going with your children is unheard of. With that love you have, you give us hope, faith, and love back every day. You do whatever it takes to ensure that none of us feel any sadness. You even wore a turkey suit last thanksgiving when we all were going through that dark time. And, yes, you did look silly in it, but we laughed for hours watching you parade around in that suit. Any man that has that much love for his family has a lot to give. It was you who got us out of our spell. It's the love you always have. It's like you always say: love is the most powerful weapon in this world, and believe me, you are armed."

"Again, I really do appreciate everything you are saying to me, but—"

"But nothing," Yolanda interrupts. "March over there and ask her out."

"I just can't right now. Besides, we have to go pick up Aunt Ruthie. Okay soldiers, everyone all set?"

"I am, Daddy, with these shoes!"

"I am glad sweetie. Gabriel?"

"I have my Pudgies!" he says with excitement.

"Okay, buddy. Whatever makes you smile. And you, princess?"

"Pretty!"

Michael smiles. "As long as you are smiling, princess."

"You see, Michael? That is exactly what I am saying—you do whatever can to make everyone smile."

At that moment, Jessica walks up. "Hi, did everyone find everything they needed?"

"Yes, Jessica, and thank you again for the advice. My daughter over here wanted me to dress like DJ something."

"It's El Mas Sin Cero, Daddy!"

"Yes, whoever that is."

Jessica smiles at Michael. "You don't get out much, do you?"

"To be honest we are only here so I can lose the frat boy image I have going on and so we can waste time while our aunt is at her magic land."

"Magic land?"

Michael whispers to her, "Doctors office."

"Oh, I'm sorry."

"No, it's okay. Everyone is strong."

"Everyone?"

"I apologize. It's a long story."

"Well, I would love to hear about it sometime."

"Really—it's nothing."

"No, honestly. I would love to hear about it. I am free tonight. Maybe we could talk about it over dinner or something."

"Well…"

"I don't mean to impose."

"No, you're fine. I just…"

"Well, I will give you my number and if you are up to it, we can talk and you can tell me your story."

"That's very flattering, and please don't take this wrong. It's just—"

Yolanda jumps in. "Yes, he will take it."

"Yolanda!"

"Don't mind him. He is shy and also is free tonight as well."

"Well, here is my number. Call me so we can meet tonight."

"He will call you soon. Thank you—you have no idea how helpful you have been today."

"Great! I guess I will see you tonight, and you can test out the blue shirt."

"Thank you."

"Okay, bye everyone."

"Bye!" say the children, waving.

"Yolanda, what were you thinking?"

"What? She is an attractive woman with a great personality, and she apparently goes after what she wants. I don't see the problem."

"It's just...who is that interested in hearing someone's story? Especially mine?"

"You're an idiot. You are acting just like a man. You are only seeing what you want to see and not knowing what is going on behind the curtain. Let's go, cuties. Everyone get your stuff together."

"Okay, Aunt Yolanda," the children say cheerfully with their things.

"Wait a minute. What just happened?"

"A blessing in disguise, Michael."

They then make it to the registers to find a cheerful cashier. "Hi, did you all find everything you needed?"

"Oh yes. We definitely found something we needed," Yolanda says, laughing.

"I am glad to hear that you all had a great experience with us today. Your total is $225.59."

"Okay, here is my card."

"If it is chipped, sir, you can just insert the card."

"I apologize. My mind is somewhere else."

Yolanda smiles. "Yeah, it is."

"Yolanda!"

"Okay, here is your receipt. Thank you for shopping with us today. Enjoy the rest of your day."

"Okay, thank you."

"Daddy… never mind."

"Sweetie, never hold back. If you have something on your mind, then say it. Don't ever be afraid to speak your mind, no matter who you are talking to. Just remember to be respectful because you are a lady."

"You need to get out more. That lady in there was nice and mommy went home."

"What are you trying to say?"

"We love you, and it's okay to have a friend. That's all I am trying to say."

Yolanda laughs. "You tell him Annabelle. It sounds like I have a cosigner."

"I love you all, but what am I going to do with you guys? Let's go pick up Aunt Ruthie."

Chapter 4

"Hey, Aunt Ruthie. How is my favorite old lady doing?"

"Tired. They gave me every shot and test they could think of."

"Yeah, that will do that to you. Let's get you home."

"Sounds good to me."

"Okay soldiers, time to go home. Goodbye Teresa. Thank you."

"Bye guys. Be safe."

"I am thinking healthy lasagna for dinner tonight. What do you guys think?"

"Okay," the children say happily.

"Yolanda?"

"That sounds good to me, Michael."

"Aunt Ruthie?"

"I am tired. I just want to crawl in my bed and sleep."

"Okay Aunt Ruthie, I will get you home."

They then head home.

"Okay soldiers, I am going to get dinner started. Go ahead do whatever it is you do on those electronics of yours. Princess, Daddy will put on the television for you."

"Yay!"

"There you are, princess. Annabelle, here is the tablet. I logged you in."

"Thank you, Daddy."

"Buddy you can either play with your toys or watch television with your sister."

"Okay."

Michael prepares dinner.

"Aunt Ruthie, I know you are tired, but you must eat something."

"I'm not hungry, Michael."

"I know you're not, but at least put something in your stomach. Here, how about a fruit bowl? I have it prepped for you in the fridge."

"How can I say no to you? Go ahead give it here."

"Thank you, Aunt Ruthie. Here you are. It's fresh."

"Thank you, Michael."

"You're welcome. I just care about your wellbeing."

"I know you do. Thank you."

"So, did Doctor Johnson say anything?"

"Yeah, the usual stuff. Watch what I eat, exercise, keep track of my sugar levels. You know…the usual doctor stuff."

"Well, he did go to school for that, so I would listen to him."

"Yeah, yeah."

"Did you tell him about you not feeling well when you woke up this morning?"

"Yes."

"What did he say?"

"It was probably because of my blood pressure."

"Really? I didn't know that can cause you to feel ill like that."

"Yeah, he said to watch my intake because high blood pressure can cause nausea."

"Well, we must monitor it closely then."

"I have that machine he gave me a while back. He wants me to keep logs of my readings."

"Well, that is what we will do then. I guess add that to the list."

She smiles at Michael. "I knew I shouldn't have told you."

"Well you know I would have called Teresa anyway."

"You're sweet for caring."

"Of course I do, my old lady."

They both share a laugh.

"You're lucky I love you so much. I am done eating. I am going to my room to get my readings from all those machines I have."

"Okay, Aunt Ruthie. I am going to get dinner out and feed my soldiers. If you need anything, let me know. Yolanda is back there as well if you need something."

"Okay, Michael. Dinner does smell good."

"There is plenty. If you want, I can set you a plate." "No, it's okay. If I get hungry, I know where to go."

"Okay, Aunt Ruthie. Remember to read a scripture and say a prayer."

"I always do."

As she walks away, Michael gets dinner out and portions it.

"All right, soldiers. I want a formation around the table."

"Coming!" says Gabriel, running.

"Daddy, let me finish this video please."

"Sweetie, you know the drill. We all eat together as a family."

"Okay, I'm coming."

"Thank you, sweetie. Princess, come get in your chair."

"'Kay!"

"There you are, princess. Let me lock you in."

"Food!"

"In a minute, princess. Hey sis, dinner is ready!"

"I'm coming, Michael."

"Did Aunt Ruthie do her logs?"

"Yes, but she is drained from her visit today, so she went to lie down."

"Is she okay?"

"Yea, you know how those shots get to some people."

"Trust me I know what that is like with these guys. Okay soldiers, looks like it is going to be us five. Who wants to say grace?"

"I will, Daddy."

"Okay buddy, go ahead and start when you are ready."

"Lord, thank you for this yummy food that we are about to eat, and thank you for us eating as a family. In Jesus' name we pray, Amen."

"Amen. Buddy, good job. Okay, let us eat. Wow, it does smell good if I don't say so myself. Oh, let me get your juices. Here you guys are. Everyone enjoying their meals?"

"Yup!" say the children with their mouths full.

"More cheese please!"

"Okay buddy, here you are."

"Thank you."

"You're welcome, buddy."

"Cheese!"

"Princess, you have a mountain of cheese on your plate. I can't even see your plate. Finish that and I will give you more."

"'Kay."

"How is the food, Yolanda?"

"It actually is pretty good. Normally I don't go for this healthy stuff, but I like it."

"See? Give things a try and if you don't like it, at least you tried. Right soldiers?"

"That's right, Daddy!" yells the children.

"Okay everyone, go ahead and continue eating. I am going to go check on Aunt Ruthie. Yolanda can you please keep an eye on them?"

"Sure, no problem."

"Excuse me, soldiers." He then proceeds to Aunt Ruthie's room.

"Hey, Aunt Ruthie, how are you feeling?"

"Drained."

"Okay, I will let you get some rest."

"Wait, Michael, I need to talk to you."

"Sure. What's going on?"

"I am okay, but it's you that we all are worried about."

"Me?"

"Yes, you. Now please listen to me. Yolanda told me about your encounter at the store today."

"She would tell you about that."

"No, listen. We are sick, yes, but you are the one feeling the pain, sorrow, and remorse."

"Aunt Ruthie, what are you talking about? Are you sure you are feeling okay?"

"Yes, I am fine, but you need to go call this girl."

"I just can't. What with the kids and now you?"

"Don't use us as an excuse."

"I apologize if it sounds like I am because I'm not. Like I told Yolanda at the store, my biggest fear is leaving you guys alone and something happens. I'm even afraid to go to the mailbox without that fear lingering. Do you understand?"

"Michael, it's like this. We are sick. Especially those babies of yours. There is nothing that is going to change that. We will be here whether it is in the physical or spiritual form."

"Please don't talk like that. I hate to even think about it."

"My point is this. Look at you. You hardly sleep, and you're constantly on guard duty as you call it. Let me ask you something. When was the last time you watched sports?"

"Sports are not my priority right now, you guys are."

"You love sports."

"Yes, this is true, but I don't have the mental capacity to watch. I am constantly on guard."

"See? That is what I am saying, Michael. Go out tonight, and for once, live your life."

"Aunt Ruthie, you guys are my life. Besides, I am just trying to guarantee that you guys have life left to live in you all."

"You can't. I am sorry to be blunt, but you just can't. As you already know this personally, there are no guarantees in life. Look. Sometimes you must gamble at life and go all in. If you are interested in this girl, then go call her."

"First, I will never gamble with any of your lives, and second, I feel like I will be cheating on Anna."

"I understand how you feel. When I lost my husband, your uncle, I thought, *How I can survive without him? How can I love again?* It was at that time at my lowest point that you invited me into your home with open arms. The love you have for your family… you gave me that back. You showed me the power of love; the same love God has for us all."

"I wouldn't say the same as God, but I do love you guys with all my heart."

"You're missing my point. God loves us so much that he brought us together as a family to love one another as he does. He gave you this family to show you that. As you always tell us, with hope, faith, and love we can defeat anything. He put that into you to show us that that is true. I know you feel the way you do about Anna, but she is home now. She is in good hands, and knowing her, she wouldn't want to see you this way. So, go get your children ready for bed, and go out there and enjoy yourself for once. I see the pain you have in your eyes. I would love to see happiness in them again."

"I am happy."

"You can't lie to me, and you definitely can't lie to God. I know I am no-where near as good as God is, but I see the pain in you. He sees you as you are; there is no hiding from Him. Maybe He thought you could use a friend right now. As they say, God works in mysterious ways. No, I am not saying go out and start a relationship. Just go out tonight and talk. That's all you must do. No one is forcing you into it, but Yolanda is right. Take it from someone with experience in that department; it isn't healthy for you not to move on. It has been two years. You might not think this, but you are ready to meet someone. You have a big heart please don't let it go to waste. I am going to bed now. Please listen to everything I just told you, and go out and enjoy yourself even if it's just for one night."

"Okay, Aunt Ruthie. I love you. Goodnight."

"Goodnight, Michael. I love you too."

Michael shuts the door and has a thought to himself. *Am I ready for this? Anna forgive me, but give me a sign you are okay with this. You were my one and only. I can never look at another the way I looked at you.*

He then walks into the dining room.

"Get ready, Michael."

"What? "Here is your phone. Go and call her."

Michael laughs.

"What?"

"Nothing. I guess it's perfect timing. I was just thinking about it. I was sort of praying for a sign, and then you said that. It's just funny how things work out."

"Well these cuties are almost done eating. So, do your bedtime routine that you love so much and then give her a call."

"Okay, I give up. You guys win. Hey soldiers, is everyone good and full?"

"Yes, Daddy. It was yummy."

"I am glad you said that, buddy. See, soldiers? Eating healthy isn't so bad. You know those meanies in you love fat and grease, so we must balance out meals for you guys. Don't get me wrong, Daddy loves his burgers, but if you guys have to eat healthy, then so do I."

"If healthy tastes like this, then I'm okay with it."

"Yes, sweetie it does. But truth time. Daddy hated the thought of eating healthy. That was until mommy would trick me and cook stuff like veggie pasta for spaghetti."

"Spaghetti!" yells Gabriel.

"That's right, buddy. I remember one time when mommy made cauliflower pizza and waited until I said that it was delicious. She laughed and then told me what it was."

"Mommy got you, Daddy!"

"That she did, sweetie. She knew what she was doing."

"I miss Mommy."

"Me too, Daddy," say Annabelle and Gabriel sadly.

"I know, soldiers, but Mommy didn't go anywhere. She is with us now."

"She is? Where?"

"Buddy look at what you are eating. That is her doing. I believe she knew and wanted this for us."

"What do you mean she is here, Daddy?"

"Sweetie, feel your heart."

"Okay."

"You feel it beating?"

"Yes, but it does that. Doesn't it?"

"Yes, but feel the warmth of it. The love of your family. Do you feel it?"

"Yes, a little."

"Sweetie, what I am trying to say to you all is that mommy is with us in the sense of the love she has for us. She loves us so much that that was her goal in life. To love one another as Aunt Ruthie just reminded me that God loves us. To be a family. And what are we?"

"Family!" yell the children.

"That's right, soldiers. We will always be family, no matter what happens. Understand this. Life will get hard and you will feel the pressure from it, but always remember that you are never alone. If you have the love of your family, nothing can stop you. I know I say this a lot, but love is the most powerful weapon in this world. See, that is what I mean by Mommy is here. She is the love that brought this family together. If you need a shoulder to cry on, then one is always here for you. If you need an ear to talk to or just vent, then one is always here for you. Soldiers always look out for each other. Love one another. The love you carry and have for your family is the most sacred gift from God. With that, there is nothing in this world that can stop you."

"I love you, sissy."

"I love you, bubby."

"We love you, Jazzy!"

"Love you."

"Aunt Yolanda, we love you!"

"I love you guys too."

"Daddy we love you!"

Michael is filled with emotions and tears start to fill his eyes. "I will always love you guys. You all are my inspiration. I am sorry, soldiers, I will be back."

"Michael, are you okay?"

"I am, Yolanda. It's just… I'm sorry. I can't stop crying for some reason."

"It's okay. That was very powerful. Thank you for that." Yolanda's tears begin to fall. "Look what you have done. Now I'm crying."

"Yolanda look at them. That is the definition of love."

"I can't take it anymore. Where are the tissue?"

Michael smiles. "In the bathroom, sis. I'm sorry. I am going to make that call now."

As Yolanda wipes her tears, she says, "Okay, go call her."

"Lord, thank you for moments like these and for blessing me with such a loving family. You know I feel guilty for this, but I could you use a friend to talk to. Okay, here goes nothing." Michael inputs Jessica's number and nervously waits.

"Hello?"

"Hi, it's Michael. You know... the guy without fashion sense."

"Oh yes, I remember who you are. I'm glad you called. Are you still free tonight?"

"I am, and I was wondering if you would like to meet for dinner."

"Don't judge me, but I haven't eaten yet, hoping you would call. I'm sorry... I don't know why I just told you that."

They both laugh.

"No, it's okay. I haven't eaten either. I had dinner with my family, but I spent most of the time with my aunt."

"Great! Where were you thinking of meeting at?"

"How about Ethan's Steakhouse?"

"Perfect. Will 8 o'clock work for you?"

"I am going to get my little soldiers ready for bed, and yes, 8 o'clock works for me."

"Okay, I will meet you in the lobby. See you soon. Bye!"

"Sounds good. I will see you then. Bye."

Michael goes back to the dining room.

"All right, soldiers. Line up for your medicines. Gabriel, here is yours, buddy."

"Thank you."

"Please take all of them."

"Okay."

"Annabelle here is yours, and please don't drop them."

"Okay, thank you."

"You're welcome, sweetie. Princess, here is yours. I have your juice for you take them."

"Thank you."

"You're welcome, princess. I want to see empty little cups when you are done."

"I took mine, Daddy! See?"

"Good job, buddy."

"Me too, Daddy! See?"

"Good job, sweetie."

"All gone!"

"I see that, princess. I am proud of you all. Okay soldiers. Ready to not be so stinky?"

"Daddy!" yell the children.

"Okay, princess, you're first!"

"Ducky!"

"Yes, princess, your ducky is in there waiting for you. Let's go."

"'K."

He takes her and cleans her up.

"See? All better. You smell all clean."

"Daddy princess!"

He smiles at her. "You will always be Daddy's princess. Okay, buddy, you're up. Get to it!"

"Coming!"

"Okay, princess, here is your goodnight bear. Let me tuck you in. There you are, princess. Now you are all set for sweet dreams. I know you don't know many bedtime prayers, so Daddy is going to say one for you. Okay?"

"'K."

"O heavenly father, thank you for blessing me with such a beautiful princess. As you watch over her through the night, allow her to wake at the first sight of light. In Jesus' name we pray. Amen."

"Amen."

"I love you. Goodnight!"

"Love you, Daddy."

He shuts the door as Gabriel runs up to him. "All clean, Daddy!"

"Buddy, that was fast. Are you sure you are clean?"

"Yup. Look! No stinky."

"Okay, buddy, if you say so. Let's get you into bed. Annabelle, the bathroom is free!"

"Okay, Daddy!"

"All right, buddy, monster check. Nope, not in the closet. Nope, not under the bed. Looks like you are set for night-night. Ready to say the bedtime prayer?"

"Yup."

"Okay, we will say it together."

"Now I lay me down to sleep, I pray the lord my soul to keep. Angels watch me through the night and wake me with the morning light. Amen."

"Okay. Lights out, buddy. I love you. Goodnight."

"I love you too, Daddy. Goodnight."

Michael shuts the door halfway. "Sweetie, are you good?"

"Yes. I am all clean and ready for bed."

"Okay sweetie. In your bed you go. I know you grew up on me so fast, so I guess no more monster checks."

"You can still tuck me in."

"Well, thank you. I will take you up on your offer. It will be my pleasure. Are you ready for your bedtime prayer?"

"Yes. I like Psalm 4:8. Can I say it?"

"Of course, sweetie."

"In peace I will both lie down and sleep; for you alone, o Lord, make me dwell in safety."

"Amen, sweetie. You're my big girl. How are you feeling?"

"I'm good. My medicine is making me sleepy now."

"Okay, sweetie, rest those beautiful eyes of yours. I love you. Goodnight."

"Goodnight, Daddy. I love you too."

Michael shuts the door and then heads into the kitchen.

"Yolanda what are doing?"

"Cleaning up this mess."

"That's okay I will take care of it."

"I have this handled Michael. Go get dressed."

"Okay, if you insist."

"Wear something nice."

"I hear you." He makes his way to his room and struggles in thought. *Man, what do I wear? Why is this so hard? I've never had an issue with what to wear. Okay, I am overthinking this. Just relax and take a step back. Okay, that's better. You know what? This blue shirt looks like a winner. Yes, I think I will go with this.* He gets cleaned and dressed. *Should I put on cologne? Why not? I tell the kids all the time 'no stinky.' Wait... note to self: do not talk kid-language to Jessica.*

He makes his way to Yolanda.

"You look good, Michael. And you smell good, too. Is that cologne I smell?"

"What? I like smelling good."

"If you say so. Anyways, Michael, I have some advice for you. Just be yourself tonight. You are an excellent person to be around. She is lucky."

"Hey, slow down. I wouldn't go that far. I just want a friend to talk to."

"So that explains the cologne then?"

They both laugh.

"Okay, you got me on that one. But seriously, I am not looking for someone in that type of way. I should be back right after dinner. It shouldn't be more than hour."

"Michael seriously. We will be okay here."

"It's just the kids and now Aunt Ruthie."

"I am sorry, but I worry about them."

"They are good. Everyone took their meds, and I bet they are fast asleep now. I have this under control. So, go out tonight and enjoy yourself, and do not come back in an hour. Do you hear me?"

"Okay, understood. But listen—my cell phone is on. If for any reason you need me, do not hesitate to call."

"Like I said, Michael. I have this under control. Now please go out there and enjoy yourself."

"Okay Yolanda. And thank you again. I will see you soon."

Chapter 5

"Hi Michael."

"Oh, hi Jessica. You're early. I apologize, I just didn't expect you to be here so early."

"My father always says early is on time and on time is late."

Michael smiles. "Let me guess… your father—is he a military man?"

"Yes. How did you know that?"

"I have a marine cousin, another cousin who is in the Army, and my brother is in the Army, as well."

"Wow. Patriotic, are we?"

They both laugh. "Yes, maybe just a little. Should we get a table?"

"Yes, please! I am starving."

They make their way inside and are greeted by a hostess.

"Hi. Welcome to Ethan's Steakhouse. Party of two?"

"Yes please."

"Okay right this way."

"Ladies first."

"Why, thank you, Michael."

The hostess walks them to their table. "Here you are. Your waiter will be with you momentarily."

"Okay thank you. Jessica allow me to get your chair for you."

"Thank you."

"Forgive me, but I must comment on how beautiful you look."

"That is sweet of you to say, and if you don't mind me saying so, you look handsome. I see you went with the blue shirt."

They share a laugh.

"Of course, I didn't know what to wear so I just went with your suggestion."

"It was a good choice. You look good in it."

"Thank you. So, how long have you worked at the store?"

"I have been there for two years now. Ever since I came down from Colorado Springs."

"That's interesting. Let me ask you this—is Fan Zone still open?"

She smiles. "Actually, it is. How do you know about Fan Zone?"

"My brother was stationed there."

"He was?"

"Yes. When I went to visit him years ago, I instantly fell in love with Colorado Springs. It's so peaceful there. There is so much beauty in that city."

"So, I see you're a romantic at heart."

Michael smiles. "No, I wouldn't say that, but I truly feel that you can find beauty everywhere."

"So, what is your definition of beauty?"

"I walked into that one, didn't I?"

They both share a laugh.

"I am just curious because of the way you say beauty is everywhere."

"That's fair. Well, for me, I feel that beauty is of God's creation. It is in everything we see, touch, hear, and smell. For an example, the peacefulness of snow falling. How the ocean when calm is so peaceful, and in the sunset, as well. As you watch it go down, it kisses everything in sight as if it is saying goodnight. See, that, to me, is true beauty."

"Wow. I've never heard it explained that way before."

"It is in all of us, as well."

"Us?"

"Yes, every person has true beauty in them, as well, but as you explained to me earlier how fashion is deceiving, so is beauty."

"Interesting. How so?"

"For an example, what do most people try to look like?"

"From my experience at the store, basically what is on television."

"Exactly. So, is that beauty or generated?"

"Well, generated obviously."

"That is my point. You can have thousands of dollars of work done to create beauty based on social standards, but it's not true beauty. Every one of us is beautiful just the way we are. God created us in his image. So, who are we to say that who we are isn't good enough? To say God must have made a mistake?"

"Well, I would think not."

"Exactly. He created us as we are and those who realize it are at peace knowing that we were created perfect just the way we are."

"You really put some thought into this, didn't you?"

"Forgive me for trying to sound like I am trying to change the world, but it just frustrates me to see people being told they don't meet certain standards. How we look, dress, and act isn't good enough. On the internet, in movies, on television, and even in books, there are certain requirements of how to fit in. On that, I say fit in to what? Who decided that who we are isn't good enough? I just want someone to finally stand up and say that you don't need to fit into their clubs. If they don't accept you the way you are, then so what? You don't need them because we all are in the greatest club of all—under the grace of God. And believe me, he accepts us just the way we are. If you can realize that, if you can look in the mirror and say out loud, 'I am beautiful,' then that right there, Jessica, is true beauty."

"I agree with you on that. Someone needs to let the world know that enough is enough. Trust me. I see it all the time at the store."

"I apologize for my rant."

"No, you're fine. I am blown away that someone can take what beauty is supposed to be and what it is. To be honest with you, I am impressed by it."

The waiter then comes to the table. "Hi guys. I am sorry for being so late coming over here. As you can see, we are swamped tonight. My name is Anthony; I am your server tonight. May I start you two out with something to drink? We have great two-for-one special this evening. I can start with you, ma'am."

"I will take a diet soda please."

"And for you, sir?"

"I will have a diet as well, please."

"Okay, I will be right back with those drinks. While I get those, feel free to look over our specialty steaks menu. If you have any questions, please don't hesitate to ask."

"Thank you, Anthony."

"Thank you. So, you don't drink?"

Michael smiles. "I used to drink, but when you have an army at home, that goes out the window."

"I understand that. I will have a glass of wine now and then but nothing to write home about."

"Speaking of home, I must go check in, if you don't mind."

"No, please, by all means."

"Thank you. I will only be a second."

"I will be here."

Michael excuses himself and goes to call Yolanda.

"Hello?"

"Hey Yolanda, how is the fort?"

"Did you leave her at the table to call me?"

"Yes. I just wanted to check in and see if everyone was okay."

"Michael, hang up the phone. We are fine. Bye."

"But seriously—"

"But nothing. You never leave a date alone at the table under any circumstance."

"Last time, Yolanda, it isn't a date."

"Goodbye, Michael."

"Fine. Call me if, for any reason, you need me. Goodbye." He makes his way back to the table. "I am sorry about that."

"It's no problem. The waiter brought our drinks and said he will be back in a moment."

"Okay, great."

"So, 'fort?' 'Soldiers?' You have to let me in on that."

Michael smiles. "It's a long story."

"That is one of the reasons we are here, right? I am all ears."

The waiter comes to the table and interrupts them. "Okay, folks, are we ready to order?"

"I believe so. Are you ready, Jessica?"

"Yes. I will have the sirloin—medium—with broccoli and the vegetable mix please."

"Excellent choice, ma'am. And for you, sir?"

"I will have the parmesan-crusted steak with mashed potatoes and broccoli, please."

"How would you like that cooked?"

"Oh, I am sorry. Medium-well please."

"Sounds good. I will have that out in a bit for you guys."

"Okay, thank you."

"Thank you, Anthony."

"I am impressed."

"Okay, I will bite. What are you impressed by?"

"The fact that you ordered exactly what you wanted. Most people order the minimum when meeting someone for the first time."

"I know people like that, and I really don't understand why they do it. It's as if they are trying to make a good impression or something. To me when they do that, it is a false sign immediately, because nothing impresses me more than someone who shows me their true self."

"I agree. You don't know how many times I would meet someone for the first time, and they would order salads. Not because they wanted it, but it would somehow impress me. I never understood that. It's funny, though, because later I would find out they stopped at Burger Town on the way home."

Jessica bursts into laughter. "I am sorry, but that was funny because my sisters used to do that all the time."

"So, you have sisters?"

"Yes. I have two. One is happily married with two of my beautiful nephews and the other is 15." So, your father, the military man, raised three daughters? He must have had fun."

She smiles. "Oh yes, he did. And believe me, he had his work cut out for him."

"I bet. And your mother?"

"She is amazing. She is the glue that holds us together. She is the one who instilled faith and love to us. She always told us that faith and love are the true foundation to a family."

"I couldn't agree more. She does sound like an amazing woman."

"That she is. How about you? I know about your military side but your mother, father?"

"Well, growing up, Dad had to work a lot, you know, to keep food on the table and a roof over our heads, so it was pretty much my mother, brother, sister, and me growing up. My mother, Sally, was my rock. I could go to her with any problem, and she would always speak in such a way that she would put any problems I had into simple context. I found it interesting that you say your mother talked about family. It must be a mother thing to teach their children about family because my mother was the same way. She would always tell us that family is the most important thing to have in this world, and without it, you're missing out."

"What about those without family?"

"See that is the amazing thing. She taught us that blood isn't an automatic ticket into the family club. She would always say family is someone you can count on. Someone to talk to. To laugh, cry with. Regardless of if you share genes with that type of person. She will tell us that if you share those traits with someone, then that is family."

"I like that because I have some great friends with those traits like what you just described, and they are closer to me than some of my blood family."

"That is a beautiful thing to have. My mother was also very religious. She loved church. It didn't even matter the religion. If Jesus was in your heart, she would go to any church with you. Don't even get me started on Bible groups. With my father working all the time, it was basically her and three kids, so she would host them at our house to make sure we were paying attention. On the matter of church, though, she would drag us down there every Sunday, Easter, Christmas—basically, any event that was going on, we were there."

Jessica smiles. "Yes, believe me I know what that is like. With my father being in the military, we moved from base to base. The first thing my mother would do when we arrived is find a church and join a Bible study. If there wasn't one on the base, she would establish one."

"That's interesting. Sounds like our mothers would have made good friends."

"Probably. So, when did you start to actually have faith and believe in the word?"

"I always had faith and believed. It became strong when I met my wife, but after she passed…"

"I'm sorry. I didn't mean to—"

"No, it's okay. Our faith was being tested before she passed, as well. My oldest, Annabelle, was diagnosed with progeria, which is an extremely rare genetic disorder that they say has a life expectancy of 13 years. What confuses me is that neither of us have it. The explanation we received was that it was caused by one or more abnormalities in the genome. Something about a mutation in a single gene."

"How old is she?"

"She is 12. About to turn 13."

"Michael, I don't know what to say."

"No, you're fine."

"But your other kids... are they okay?"

"Not in the medical sense. My little buddy, Gabriel, who is 10 years old, has what the doctors think is Desmoplastic Small-Round-Cell tumor or DSRCT for short. From what I read online, it is a type of cancer that is usually found in the abdomen, but it can also occur in other parts of the body. His doctor is one of the best, and he suspects that that is what he is suffering from and is giving him treatments for it. He had surgery recently for it. I pray that is not what he has, because by the time DSRCT is diagnosed, it would have spread to his liver, lymph nodes, lungs, or bones. We get the test results back soon to confirm it."

"What about your youngest child?"

"Yes, Jazmyn, my princess. She is 3 years old. She was diagnosed with neuroblastoma, which is a rare cancer. It's in her kidneys. That is why she has a lump in her neck. So that she doesn't feel self-conscious about it, we call it her little bubble. My wife never lost faith, and she would tell us all never give up on God or ourselves. That he has a plan. Then, when she passed, it was up to me to carry that mindset on."

"Oh my lord, Michael. How? I apologize I am trying to come up with words, but I seem not to be able to."

"Don't worry. It is like learning something new for the first time. Your brain must adjust.

"You tell me so calmly though."

"It's not that, because believe me, my brain never shuts down for what they call normal activities. To be honest with you, I was hesitant about coming here tonight."

"Michael if you need to leave, I completely understand."

"No offense, but I tried to stay home. My sister talked me into it and assured me that everything will be okay at home. So here I am."

"I am just speechless about everything you told me about your children and wife."

"I apologize for that. I gave you a lot to process."

"Well, to be honest. Yes, you did. I wouldn't know what to do if I were in your situation. I would call every doctor, nurse, basically anybody with a license for help."

"There is one thing about that. Yes, I am dependent on the medical field, but I have something stronger than medicine. I have faith. You see I am not calm or scared. I am in the middle. I will do whatever it is the Lord asks of me to heal my family. So, I must remain calm and trust in the Lord. I must be what we call in my family the general. I cannot show an ounce of fear. My little soldiers are scared and hurting every day. So, I must be the one that encourages them to stay strong."

"So, is that where the military language comes from?"

"Well, yes. It's like this. I tell them that they are soldiers out in the battlefield of life. With meanies—meaning cancer—trying to attack them. I tell them that they have three things that will help them through it. Hope, faith, and love. Allow me to explain it in military terms. With hope they can make it through the battlefield. Faith, as in their armor, is always protecting them. Finally, we have love, their weapon against any enemy they come across. With those three things, they can defeat anything that goes up against them."

"I like that. So, what is your outlet?"

"Outlet?"

"Yes. What do you do to get away from it all?"

"They are my outlet. They go through this day in, day out, and yet stay as one. Yes, they cannot just go play outside or go the park, but my children are so strong they make what they have a part of their lives. You know, there are some people who hear what they have and start to feel sorry for them. Please don't get me wrong, I appreciate the gesture, but my children don't need sympathy like that because in their eyes they are not sick. It is just part of their lives. They are so strong, they take these illnesses and run with it. Of course, I would love to take them to a water park or zoo, but they love their lives because we have each other. We do go to a special place all the time. It is sort of a theme park called Adventure Land."

"Adventure Land? I don't think I ever heard of that park."

"It is the cancer center."

"Why is the cancer center called Adventure Land?"

"We call it that because you never know what we will encounter there. The kids at first were afraid of going there, so I told them it is a land of adventure—a magical place where sickness goes away. They can be themselves there. Besides, I couldn't say, 'Hey, soldiers, we are going to the Tampa Cancer Center today.' So, Adventure Land was born."

"I understand now."

"We also call their treatments magic potions."

"Magic potions?"

"Yes, because I cannot tell them, 'Let's get you ready for chemotherapy or radiation therapy.' I want them to feel comfortable and just be children."

"That is cute. It does make sense to me."

"I also told them it is a theme park because the staff is one of the best in the world. They dress up in silly costumes for the children. They bring in cartoon characters. Even athletes stop by just to say hi to all the children. It is indescribable to see the look on all the children's faces when things like that happen. Unfortunately, some children are in such agony, but when they get to have experiences like what I just described, even if it is for a second, it is amazing to see them smile. They get so happy that it's as if, for just that moment, all the illnesses they suffer from go away and they turn into normal children."

"That must be amazing to see. I like the way you guys turned it into a theme park. It is as if you created an escape world for your children."

"Thank you, but to be honest with you, I should not get the credit for it. I only told my children it is Adventure Land. It is the staff, those who stop by to be with the children, and those who donate to fund all the activities and to fund research to find cures. All of those people who are involved… they are the ones who deserve the credit for making Adventure Land what it is. Without those people, it is just a gloomy hospital. To me, all the children in hospitals around the world are the strongest force in the world. They all are real inspirations. All those children, including mine, have these illnesses and don't show any weakness because they all carry hope, faith, and love.

"I see people every day who go through their lives, then when something bad happens, they are quick to give up on their hopes and dreams because they say life isn't fair. I want to tell those people to try living through an I.V. for once. Try hearing that you may have a year left to live. You see, Jessica, all the children in hospitals like Adventure Land have these illnesses and do what a lot of us take for granted. They cherish every minute they have. They get diagnosed with what they have, but they are strong and never give up. It is just amazing to see that."

"Wow! You are so passionate about everything you said. I understand now why you gave me the definition of beauty earlier. I will be honest with you, I feel guilty now."

"Why do you say that? It isn't your fault or anyone's. It is just a part of God's plan. It's not for us to understand his plan. But I will tell you this: speaking for my family, giving up is not an option."

"No, I feel guilty because just the other day, I lost my favorite earrings and all I could say was, 'Why do bad things happen to me?'"

They both laugh.

"No, I didn't mean for you to feel bad. It's just that, when you have a family like I do, you see life in a different way."

"I bet. After hearing everything you just said, I will look at life differently, as well."

"Wow, we finished. I don't even remember the waiter bringing our meals to us."

"Neither do I."

"That is weird. Normally, I am very observant. Now that I look around, the restaurant seems to be empty."

Jessica smiles. "I guess the world disappears on us sometimes."

"I'm sorry?"

"I was just saying, you know how sometimes it feels like you are in a different place and you don't notice the world around you? Did I say something wrong?"

"I apologize. You just reminded me of something."

The waiter then comes to the table. "So, did you guys enjoy your meals? I would have said something earlier, but you two seem to be having an interesting conversation."

Michael and Jessica both smile.

"I am sorry about that, but yes, everything was delicious."

"It must have been delicious. We both finished our meals and didn't even notice."

They all share a laugh.

"I am glad to hear you both enjoyed your meals. May I interest you two in dessert?"

"I think I am good on dessert. Jessica how about you?"

"No, I am okay. Thank you."

"Allow me to take your plates from you two, and I will leave you the check here on the table. We are closing soon. There is no rush. Whenever you are ready, I will be happy to take it up for you."

Jessica reaches for the check. "I will take care of the check."

"It's okay, Jessica, I will take care of it."

"I don't mind, Michael. After all, it was my idea to come out."

"I appreciate that, Jessica, and I understand that in this day and age things are different. I respect and admire an independent woman such as yourself, but please let me take care of dinner. It will be my treat. Besides you heard an earful from me tonight. That is payment enough."

"Well, thank you, Michael. To be honest, I loved hearing you speak."

"Here you are, Anthony."

"I will be right back with your receipt."

"Okay, thank you. You know, Jessica, I will let you in on a secret. I wouldn't be able to pick what I just ate out of a line up. I can't remember what I had eaten."

"I am glad to hear you say that because I thought I was the only one."

As they both laugh, the waiter comes back to the table. "Here you are, sir, I just need a signature, and the other copy is for you."

"Okay. Thank you. Here you are. I appreciate your services, Anthony, thank you."

"Yes, thank you, were wonderful tonight."

"I appreciate you both saying that. Please have a safe trip home."

"Okay, thank you. I still cannot believe it is closing time already. I'd better get home."

"Yes, it is getting late."

The waiter comes back to the table. "Sir, I think you made a mistake on the tip."

"No, it's correct. That is yours."

"But, sir, the bill was only $68, and you tipped me $100. I think you put too many zeros down."

"I didn't make a mistake. You were wonderful tonight. That is for you."

"Sir, I only brought your meals out."

"Sometimes that's all that it takes. You have a tough job, and I know sometimes people don't tip like they should because they think you're just bringing meals out. This is the way you are making a living, and I have to say you are a master at your craft. You made sure we enjoyed our meals and, admittedly, we didn't notice the food, but you yourself were great. You saw that we were in an important conversation and you didn't interrupt us. To that, I say thank you."

"Sir I don't know how to thank you."

"Anthony, there is a way you can thank me."

"Name it. It's done."

"Just pay it forward. If you see a homeless person, don't walk by them. Instead ask if they have eaten yet, and if not, buy them something to eat. If you see an elderly person in need of assistance, help them. Better yet, hospitals all around here need volunteers. They need people with good hearts. I know I don't know you, but you look to have a good heart to me. You were honest enough to come back and ask if I had made a mistake when most people would take it and run. God put it into my heart to give you that tip. He must have a reason."

"Sir, thank you so much."

"Thank you, Anthony."

The waiter walks away in tears.

"That was very sweet of you, Michael."

"I apologize I didn't think he was going to come back. I didn't want you to know I had tipped him that. Like I was trying to impress you."

"No, you are fine. I think it's sweet how you asked him to pay it forward and the way you said that God put it into your heart. I see how you recruit volunteers now."

Michael and Jessica both smiles.

"Are you ready to get out of here?"

"Yes."

They both get up and exit the restaurant.

"Allow me to walk you to your car."

"Yes, that is very nice of you."

"I had a great time tonight, and again, I apologize for ranting on like I did."

"You can stop apologizing. I had great time tonight. It was fun. I loved hearing the way you spoke. It was very inspiring. You are definitely different than the guys I usually meet."

"You have my curiosity. How am I different?"

"For one, you picked this place to have dinner."

"They have good steaks here."

"Most men will try to impress me and take me to Mario's or some other fine dining restaurant. Also, the way you didn't try hard to impress me. Everything you said and did impressed me. It was easy for you like it was part of your personality or something to that effect."

"It is like I tell my children all the time: just be who you are. That is the way we were created. Why be someone you are not?"

"See that is what I mean? You have a passion for even the littlest of things. Normally when I meet a guy, they ask me the usual questions. It's either *How old are you?* Or *Where did you go to college?* You know… basic information. You are just different. You have so many feelings invested in what you believe in and are not afraid to show it. To put the icing on the cake, you are a God-loving man and one who doesn't try to hide it. Which to me is high up on the impressive chart."

"I appreciate that, and you are a great person to talk to. You have such a wonderful personality; you made it easy to share with you. I just hope I didn't bring you down about my family. Normally I don't speak so freely about their conditions like it is a conversation piece or topic of discussion."

"You didn't bring me down at all. I know someone in your position will never use their children's conditions for topic of discussion or try to get sympathy points. It must have been hard for you to talk about. Especially about your wife's passing. I will be praying for you and your family's well-being."

"I thank you for keeping them in your prayers. It is very hard talking about everything that is going on with them and of my wife's passing. On the topic of my children, they need every prayer possible. They have a long road ahead of them, but with God's help, I can drive them safely onto their paths."

"That right there is a prime example of what I said earlier. You are very passionate."

"Speaking of family, I really need to head home and check in on them. I just worry so much about them when I am away for so long."

"From everything you have told me, I completely understand. I really did enjoy this evening, and thank you again for dinner."

"It was my pleasure."

"I hope to hear from you soon. You know you can call me anytime if you need someone to talk to."

"I appreciate that, and I will keep that in mind."

"I am serious Michael. With everything you have going on in your life, you're just one man. I hope you understand that you are not alone. I will always be on the other side of the phone if you need me, or we can meet for coffee sometime if you need to get out of the house."

"Thank you again for your offer. We have appointments at Adventure Land these next three days, so I will be tied up with my little soldiers, but I do like the idea of calling you."

"I am available anytime you need to talk. Time is not a factor. Even if it is late at night, I will always pick up the phone."

"You are a very special woman with a big heart. I am glad we were able to talk and have dinner together."

"As am I."

"Have a safe trip home. Goodnight."

"Goodnight Michael."

Michael then gets in his car and heads home. As he walks through the door, he looks for Yolanda. "Hey, sis, I'm home. There you are on the couch. What are you doing? Oh, you're sleeping. I am sorry, sis. Here is a blanket for you. Love you. Goodnight. Okay, let me do a quick check on everyone."

He goes and checks on the children. As he does that, he stands in the hallway looking into their rooms and says a prayer. "Look at them, Lord. Thank you for your many blessings. You gave them life. Lord please don't allow any more death to happen to this family. You have your reasons for taking Anna back, but please tell me what you want me to do to save them. Lord, please heal my children from their sufferings and allow them to live their lives as you intended. You are our father, and I know you have a plan for us all. I just need to know what I can do. Use me, Lord, as your instrument. I will gladly do what is asked of me. Thank you, Lord, for always being here for us and watching over this world. Give us the strength to carry on your word and to be who you designed us for. In your heavenly name, Jesus, I pray. Amen."

Chapter 6

The alarm clock goes off.

"Wow, 6:30 already? Oh well. Time to get up and get breakfast started before my little soldiers come out."

Michael goes out into the kitchen and starts to prepare breakfast. He, of course, hears Jazmyn. "Hi princess. Good morning. How do you feel today?"

"Sickie, Daddy."

"That is what I was afraid of, but we are going to Adventure Land today for your magic potion so you can feel better."

"'Kay."

"I am going to get your special breakfast just for you so your potion goes good with your tummy."

"Not hungry, Daddy."

"Princess, I understand that you are not feeling well, but you must eat something to allow your potion to work. Otherwise you are going to be more sickie when you leave Adventure Land. Just please try for me. Can you do that for Daddy?"

"'Kay, Daddy."

"Okay, let's get you into your chair, and I will put on your favorite cartoons just for being my big girl."

"Yay! I big girl!"

"Yes, you are, princess. Let me find your show… Okay, there you are, princess. Daddy is going to get your breakfast ready."

"'Kay."

As he does that, out come Annabelle and Gabriel. "Daddy!" they shout.

"Good morning, soldiers. Did we brush our teeth?"

"Aw, man!"

"Gabriel, you are going to learn one of these days, buddy. Please go back and get to it."

"Okay, I will." Gabriel runs off.

"I did, Daddy. See?"

"I believe you, Annabelle. Sweetie, how are you feeling today?"

"I feel okay today."

"Just okay?"

"I am good because God woke me up and that is a blessing. Right, Daddy?"

"That is right, sweetie. Always be thankful for that. You know, most people take that for granted, but God loves us so much that He gave us this day to be together."

"I know, Daddy. That is why I thanked him when I woke up."

"I am sure he appreciates it, sweetie. I am getting your sister's special breakfast ready and then I will get you and your brother's out as well. If you want, you can watch television or go on your tablet, and yes, I logged you in already."

"Okay. Thank you for that, Daddy."

"Anytime, sweetie." Michael then prepares Jazmyn's breakfast. "Okay, princess, here you are. One special breakfast for my big girl. Please drink all of it. I need you to be very strong for today."

"Thank you."

"You are very welcome." As he gets everyone else's breakfast ready, out comes Gabriel.

"All clean, Daddy. See?"

"Very good, buddy. You know, one day you must remember to brush your teeth as soon as you wake up."

"Yes sir."

"Thank you, buddy. Please sit at the table."

"Okay. I am hungry!"

"Annabelle, breakfast is ready."

"Coming!"

"Here you guys are… Who wants to say grace?"

"I will, Daddy."

"Okay, buddy. Whenever you are ready."

"What about Aunt Yolanda and Aunt Ruthie?"

"They will be out shortly. I don't want your food to get cold, so it is okay if you guys eat. Thank you for thinking of them."

"Okay. Dear Lord, thank you for this yummy food Daddy made for us to eat. And please be with Jazzy today when she gets her magic potion, so she won't feel sickie. In Jesus' name we pray. Amen."

"Amen buddy. I am proud of you for including your sister in your prayer."

"Thank you, Daddy, and I always pray for my family."

"Me too, Daddy. I pray for all of us every day."

"I am proud of both of you, and I know heaven is as well. You two—and yes, Jazzy, you as well—are perfect examples of God's children."

The children giggle.

"Listen up, soldiers. As you know, we are going to Adventure Land today for Jazzy. If you need anything at all or are not feeling well, let me know, because while we are there, I can get you checked out."

"Daddy, I said I am okay."

"Me too, Daddy."

"I apologize, soldiers, but you all know I care about you so much."

"I know you care about us, Daddy, but we will let you know if something hurts."

"Yeah, Daddy."

"Okay, soldiers. I am just making sure we are on the same page. I trust you guys."

Yolanda then comes out. "Good morning, Michael. Hi cuties."

"Good morning, Aunt Yolanda!" they shout.

"Good morning, sis. I came in, and you were fast asleep on the couch."

"Yeah, I crashed at about 10 o'clock or so I think."

"What time did you go into your room?"

"To tell you the truth, I don't even remember. What time did you come home?"

"I arrived here at maybe 11:30."

"Where did you go, Daddy?"

"Well, buddy, Daddy went out to have dinner with a friend."

"Was it that lady from the store yesterday?"

Michael smiles. "Yes, sweetie, that is who I had dinner with."

"I am glad you didn't come home within an hour, Michael."

"To be honest with you, I kind of lost track of time."

"Don't even get me started with you leaving her at the table to call me."

"Hey, you know how my mind works. I can only apologize so many times about how much I worry."

"I understand you worry, but that was a rookie move. You never do that."

Michael smiles. "Well, technically, I am a rookie."

"Okay, Michael, if you say so."

Aunt Ruthie then comes out. "Hello everyone. How are my little babies doing this morning?"

"Good!" The children shout.

"Good morning, Michael, Yolanda."

"Morning, Aunt Ruthie."

"Good morning, Aunt Ruthie. It is good to see your beautiful face today."

"You are too much, Michael."

"Breakfast is ready if both of you are hungry. I hope you don't mind that we started without you two. I didn't want the kids' food to get cold, and Jazzy needed her special breakfast for her magic potion today. She isn't feeling all that well."

Aunt Ruthie goes to Jazmyn. "Aww, my poor baby. Is you not feeling good?"

"No."

"It is okay. Aunt Ruthie is here for you, baby."

As Jazmyn goes to give her a hug, she says, "Thank you."

"Anytime, baby."

"That's right, cutie, and Aunt Yolanda is here too. Breakfast does smell good."

"It does, Michael."

"Thank you both. Please help yourselves. There is plenty."

"Thank you."

"Yes, thank you, Michael. So how did it go last night?"

"Well, sis, it went very well. I had a good time."

"So, you did go out last night, Michael?"

"I did in fact go out, Aunt Ruthie."

"That is a surprise that you took Yolanda and my advice."

He smiles. "Well, I finally gave in to both of your peer pressure."

"Whatever helps you sleep at night, Michael. Did you enjoy yourself?"

"I did, Aunt Ruthie."

"That is good to hear."

"So, where did you have dinner?"

"We ate at Ethan's Steakhouse."

"That is where you took her, Michael?"

"I did, Yolanda, and she appreciated that."

"She did?"

"Yes. She said that most guys try to take her to some fine dining, but she liked that I chose that restaurant."

"Really? Well, I for one understand where she is coming from with guys trying so hard to impress us women like they think it matters where we eat. She sounds like a good woman, and you are definitely not like most guys out there."

"You know, it is funny to hear you say that because she basically said the same thing. We had a good evening last night."

"See? I told you that you would have fun. If you don't mind me asking, what did you two talk about?"

"I don't mind it all, Yolanda. We talked about family mostly."

"You told her everything that is going on here?"

"Yes, surprisingly, I did. It was a relief to talk to someone outside this family about what is going on."

"You two were right. I guess I just needed that extra push. She has such a great personality that it was easy for me to talk to her. We talked about these soldiers and their conditions. I even talked about Anna."

"I am just surprised to hear you say that. You are usually reserved when anyone tries to talk about your children's conditions. Especially when it comes to talking about Anna."

"I agree with Yolanda on that. What possessed you to talk about topics that you are mostly guarded about?"

"Well, Aunt Ruthie, Yolanda, we first talked about family, and then we got on the topic of faith. She asked me when I started to have faith and believe in the Word of the Lord. So, I told her how I came about my faith, and I then told her how my faith started to blossom when I met Anna. I even proceeded to tell her how my faith was being tested with these soldiers' conditions. It was an interesting conversation. It's funny though. When we were done talking, it was at that point that we realized that we were done eating. We were so deep into our conversation that we hadn't realized that our waiter had brought our meals to us."

"Wow! That must have been a great conversation if you two didn't realize you were eating."

"I agree with Yolanda."

Michael smiles at them. "Like I said, it was a great evening. I really want to thank you both for kind of forcing me to go."

"You see what happens when you give people a chance, Michael? I told you at the store it was a blessing to have run into her. I am glad to hear that you had a great time with her."

"As am I."

"Thank you both, and I will admit to the fact that maybe God decided that I needed a friend at this point of my life to help me cope with everything that is going on."

"So, when do you see her again?"

"To be honest, Yolanda, I do not have the slightest clue. I am going to be extremely busy. These soldiers have appointments at Adventure Land, these next three days. So, it is up in the air right now."

"I understand that you are going to be busy with these cuties, but you can at least call her. It doesn't take that much time out of your day to call some-one—like perhaps after these cuties go to bed."

"I agree with Yolanda on that statement, Michael."

"Yes, this is true, but at this moment all my attention and focus are on my little soldiers and their well-being. Am I right soldiers?"

"That's right, Daddy!"

"You see, Yolanda? Even my little buddy agrees with me. He is my right-hand man."

"What does that mean?"

Michael laughs. "It means that you always have Daddy's back on anything I say."

"Oh yeah, I am. See sissy? I am Daddy's right-hand man!" Gabriel says with excitement as everyone laughs.

"Oh yeah, Bubby? Well, I am Daddy's big girl!"

Yolanda laughs. "Look what you started Michael."

"Okay, soldiers, settle down. Everyone is a winner; you all are very special to me. I love you all equally."

"Well, Daddy, like I said yesterday, it's okay to have a friend. So, I'm glad you had a good time last night."

"Well, thank you, sweetie."

"Me too, Daddy."

"Thank you, buddy, but it is just what I had said earlier. She is just daddy's friend."

"Yeah, cuties, at least for now." Yolanda and Aunt Ruthie both laugh.

"Okay, you two. I don't need any commentary from the peanut gallery. Anyways, it looks like everyone is finished eating. You all know what time it is."

"Medicine time?"

"That is correct, buddy. Okay, soldiers, come and get your little cups, and remember not to drop your medicines. It takes Daddy a long time to count them all out. Here you are, Annabelle."

"Thank you."

"You're welcome, sweetie. And Gabriel here is yours."

"Thank you."

"You're welcome, buddy."

"Daddy me?"

"Princess, you had yours in your special breakfast. I can't give you your regular cup because you are going to get magic potion today. Remember?"

"Yeah."

"I want to see empty cups, guys."

"All gone, Daddy."

"My cup is empty too, Daddy. See?"

"Good job, soldiers. Okay, Annabelle, Gabriel, please go get ready so we can take princess to Adventure Land."

"Okay, Daddy!" shout Annabelle and Gabriel as they run off.

"Yolanda, I am going to get Jazmyn ready to go, then I will clean all this up."

"It's okay, Michael. I will get it."

"Are you sure? You have been cleaning up a lot lately. I hate to put you in that position."

"It's no problem. I don't mind it at all."

"Okay, thank you. I appreciate all that you do around here. Aunt Ruthie, are you coming with us? If so, you must go get dressed."

"I was going to stay here and watch my shows, but I already told baby girl I am here for her, so I will go get dressed."

"You can stay if you want, Aunt Ruthie. She is just going in for her magic potion."

"No, it's okay. I will go and help Yolanda watch the babies while you go with Jazzy into the treatment room."

"Okay, Aunt Ruthie. I am sure Jazmyn would love it with you being there with us, and you are right. Yolanda probably will need a hand with Annabelle and Gabriel. You know how long treatments take, and let's be honest, children do not like waiting. Okay princess, let's go get you dressed."

"'Kay, Daddy."

He takes Jazmyn to her room and as he dresses her, she clutches her stomach. "Hurts, Daddy!"

"I know it does, princess, but like I said, we are going to Adventure Land to make you feel all better."

Jazmyn starts to cry. "Daddy, hurts!"

"Princess, what hurts?"

"Tummy!"

"Okay, we are going in now." With worry in his voice, he shouts to Yolanda. "Hey Yolanda!"

She comes running. "Yes Michael?"

"Without causing any panic, please make sure the children and Aunt Ruthie are dressed and ready to leave as soon as possible. We are going to Adventure Land now. She is in a lot of pain." "What is it from?"

"That is what is scaring me. Usually on the days of their treatments, I expect them to be sick or hurting as usual because that is why they are going in for treatments. But I have never seen her in pain like this before. So many things are going through my head right now I am starting to wonder if this will happen to Annabelle and Gabriel when it's time for them to go in for their treatments."

"Okay, Michael, I will make sure everyone is dressed and ready to go."

"Thank you, Yolanda."

Yolanda then rushes everyone to get ready.

"Daddy!"

"I know, princess. I am sorry you are hurting. Daddy is hurrying up as fast as I can. Okay, princess, I have your bag, and you are dressed. Let's go." Michael, holding Jazmyn, goes to the door, shouting to everyone. "Soldiers! Yolanda! Aunt Ruthie! We must leave!"

"Michael, what is going on? Jazzy, why are you crying, baby girl?"

With tears in her eyes, Jazmyn responds, "Hurt."

"I have never seen her in this much pain, Aunt Ruthie."

"Yolanda!"

"I am coming! I just can't find my other shoe!"

Annabelle comes to the door. "Daddy, is Jazzy okay?"

"Yes, sweetie. She is just hurting from the meanies."

"Jazzy, don't worry! When you get your magic potion, those meanies will go away."

"Thank you for that, sweetie. She needs us right now."

Gabriel comes out. "I'm here, Daddy."

"Okay, buddy. Thank you for hurrying."

Gabriel sees Jazmyn crying. "What's wrong with Jazzy, Daddy?"

"She is hurting, buddy."

"Aww, Jazzy, come here, and let me give you a hug." He gives her a big hug. "It's going to be okay, Jazzy."

"That was very nice of you, buddy. Aunt Ruthie, can you get them into the car?"

"No problem. Let's go, babies."

"Thank you. Hey, sis! We must leave!"

Yolanda comes running to the door. "I am sorry, Michael. I had to get everyone ready before I did, but I am here now."

"Thank you, Yolanda, and I appreciate you getting them ready so quickly."

"You're welcome. I will lock the door. Let's go ahead and go."

"Okay, thank you."

With everyone in the car, they then head to the hospital.

"Hurts!" Jazmyn cries out loud.

"Daddy, Jazzy won't stop crying. Is she going to be okay?"

"Yes, buddy. She just needs her magic potion." With thoughts going into Michael's head, he says a prayer. *Lord, with your healing hand. Please come down and touch my princess so that she won't feel this pain she is in. Many things you have done for us already. I thank you for everything. Lord, please hear my prayer. In Jesus' name I pray. Amen.*

"Michael!"

"Yes, Yolanda, what is it?"

"Did you hear me?"

"No, what did you say?"

"I was saying that I know you are in a rush, but please watch your speed. You are driving kind of fast. You have to remember that you have a carload of people."

"I apologize. My mind was somewhere else."

"It's okay, Michael. What is going through your head right now?"

"To be honest, I wouldn't be able to say. So many thoughts are creeping into my mind that I just needed to pray for Jazmyn."

"I understand, Michael, but we will get there soon."

"I know, Yolanda, and again, I apologize for my driving."

They then arrive at the hospital.

"Adventure Land!" shout the children.

"Yes, soldiers, we are here. Everyone out of the car, and let's go inside."

They all get out of the car, walk in, and go inside to an elevator to the children's floor.

"Daddy, hurts!"

"I know, princess. Why does this elevator seem to take forever?"

"Michael, it is going to be okay. We are here now."

"I know, Aunt Ruthie, but... I am sorry."

"Don't apologize, Michael. You are a loving father. Of course you have every right to worry. I would, too, if I were in your shoes."

"Thank you, Aunt Ruthie."

They arrive on the children's floor.

"Don't worry about a thing, princess. We are here now. Let's get you checked in." Michael takes Jazmyn to the front check in desk. "Hi Stephanie."

"Good afternoon, Michael. Hi Jazmyn."

"I know we are early, but Jazmyn is in a lot of pain today. I was wondering if she can get her treatment as soon as possible."

"Of course! We definitely can get her back into the treatment area. Let me call the nurse for you and tell her she is here."

"Okay, thank you so much, Stephanie."

"It's no problem at all Michael. That is why we are here."

"Yolanda, Aunt Ruthie, Stephanie is getting her back there now. Are you two sure you will be okay with Annabelle and Gabriel?"

"For the last time, Michael, yes."

"We will take care of these babies. Just go make sure baby girl gets what she needs to feel better."

"Okay, thank you both. I honestly wouldn't know what I would do without both of your help. Yolanda, here is my card. If you two or the children get hungry, please take them down to get something to eat. They know where everything is at in this hospital. They can play in the playroom if they want. Also, here are the tablets for both."

"Okay, Michael, just take care of Jazzy. We will handle it out here."

"Yes, Michael, just worry about baby girl."

"Thanks again. Okay, soldiers, listen up. Please listen to Aunt Yolanda and Aunt Ruthie. They will be out here with you while I go back in with Jazzy. I know I don't ever have to worry about you two misbehaving, but please be good. Okay?"

"Okay Daddy!" they both say with smiles.

"Thank you, soldiers. I love you both."

"We love you too, Daddy!" The children said as they give Michael a hug.

"Jazzy, it's going to be okay."

"Yeah, you will feel all better soon."

"Don't worry. She hears you guys; she just is hurting."

The nurse then comes out. "Michael we are ready for her."

"Okay, thank you, Kayla."

"Hi Jazmyn. Are you ready for your magic potion?"

"Yes. Hurts," she cries.

"Aww, sweetie, we will get you feeling better."

"Right this way, Michael. We are set up for her."

They then head into the treatment room.

"Excuse me, Kayla. Is Dr. Lee around?"

"Yes, she is here. Do you need her for anything?"

"Yes. I was wondering if she can look at Jazmyn while she is here."

"I'm sure she wouldn't mind."

"Okay, thank you. I really appreciate that."

"It's no problem. Okay, you can lay her in the chair, Michael."

"Here you are, princess. Are you ready for your potion?"

"Yes," she says softly.

"Okay, Jazmyn. You are just going to fell a little pinch, and then your magic potion will start to work."

"Daddy!"

"I am here, princess. It's going to be okay. Look! Daddy is a gorilla." He proceeds to act like one.

"You did very good, Jazmyn, and now you will get your magic potion in you soon."

"See princess? It didn't hurt."

"Daddy funny," she says smiling.

"Anything for that smile, princess."

"Everything is going to be okay, Jazmyn. Michael, I will page Dr. Lee for you and let her know Jazmyn is back here."

"Okay, thank you so much, Kayla."

"My pleasure. Jazmyn, get comfortable, and you will feel better in no time."

"'Kay."

"She is so cute, Michael."

"Thank you. Look, princess, I brought your sickie bear."

"Yay! Sickie bear!" she says, clutching the bear.

"I almost forgot, Jazmyn. Do you want to watch cartoons?"

"Yay!"

"I apologize, Michael. Is that okay?"

"She is the boss, and you know her answer."

The nurse smiles. "They are always the boss, no matter how old they get."

"You can say that again."

"There you are, Jazmyn. You have your bear and cartoons. You should be all set up now."

"Thank you."

"You're welcome, sweetie. Michael, I already let Dr. Lee know that Jazmyn is here, and she should be back here very soon."

"Okay, thank you, Kayla."

"Look Daddy! Toons!"

"I see, princess. You know, we are going to start reading books soon, instead of all this television watching you are doing."

"No!"

"Okay, princess. You say that now, but we shall see. I want you to start learning words other than what is on the television so you can be my big girl."

"I big girl!"

"That you are, princess. You know, sissy and bubby read all the time, and they are big, as well. Yes, they get to play on their tablets and watch television, but I make sure they read every day."

"Read?"

"Yes, princess, they read books, and they even read the Bible, which soon I pray you do too."

"Jesus."

"That is right, princess. When did you get so smart?"

She giggles. "Look Daddy! Piggy!"

"I see that. What happened to the good days when cartoons were just on Saturdays? Now they are on with a click of the button. Wow, do I sound old."

"Daddy old."

Michael smiles at Jazmyn. "That I am princess. Don't worry, it will catch up to you some day. How do you feel, princess?"

"Hurts."

"Don't worry, princess, soon it will go away. I know you must be feeling better if you can call me old."

"Old daddy."

"Ha-ha, I hear you princess. Just enjoy your cartoons."

Some time goes by, then the doctor walks in. "Hi Jazmyn, what are you holding?"

"Sickie bear!"

"I see you have your bear and cartoons on. Well, we know who wears the pants in this family, right Michael?"

Michael laughs. "Guilty as charged, doctor. How are you doing today?"

"I am doing great. Thank you for asking. So, what is the problem today?"

"She is in a lot more pain than usual. I know it is supposed to be normal on treatment days like you explained to me before, but she was clutching her stomach earlier, in tears, and I really don't understand why. I am just concerned."

"It's okay to be concerned, Michael. I will look and see what, if any, the problem is."

"Thank you, doctor."

"You know, we see each other enough that I said you can call me Rebecca."

"I know you expressed that to me before many times, but I respect the fact that you went to school and worked very hard to be called doctor."

"It's only a title, Michael. I am still just like you."

"I know, but it's the principal of it. You are very good at your job and an excellent doctor."

"Well, thank you, Michael; that means a lot. Okay, Jazmyn, let's see what we have here." The doctor begins to examine Jazmyn. "I am just going to press on your tummy."

"Ouchy."

"Does that hurt?"

"Yes."

"It doesn't tickle?"

"No."

"Okay, I am going to look at your bubble. Does it hurt when I touch it like this?"

"Ouchy!"

"Okay, Jazmyn, you were a very good girl for me. I am sorry I hurt you, but I had to see where it hurts. Nurse, can you draw blood and get the results to me as soon as possible please?"

"Yes, doctor."

"What is going on?"

"I can only speculate on a theory now, and you know I don't like to do that. I will have to wait until I get her results back to either confirm or deny my suspicions. Don't worry, Michael I know what must be going through your head now, but it could just be nothing. As soon as I know something, I will let you know what I think is happening."

"Okay, doctor, but you know you are kind of scaring me a little."

"I just think it is odd that she is still in pain while she is receiving her treatment. Usually children with her condition respond well while receiving high dosage of … well, her magic potion. As I said, don't worry, Michael. I will let you know when I get the results back. Please be patient. You know that I always explain everything to help you understand her condition."

"I know that, doctor, and I trust you. Thank you."

"You're welcome, Michael. I will see you soon. Bye, Jazmyn—feel better for me."

"Bye!"

"Okay, Jazmyn, just one more pinch, I promise. I know you hate needles. I will tell you a secret: so do I."

"Daddy!"

"Princess, look! Daddy is a gorilla again. Look, see?" He then acts like one again for Jazmyn.

"Daddy funny!"

"I know he is, isn't he? Okay, Jazmyn, I am all done. You were a very good girl."

"Yay!"

"I told you, princess. You are my big girl."

"I big girl!"

"Yes, you are, but you are still my princess."

"I will be back, Michael. I am going to get these over to the lab."

"Okay, Kayla. Thank you. So, princess, I see you are feeling better. You laughed at Daddy being silly. I know I probably know the answer, but how are you feeling?"

"Sickie."

"That is what I figured you would say, princess. It just means that your magic potion is working. Don't worry. When you are all done, we will get home, and you can get some rest. Then, tomorrow, you can terrorize your brother and sister. Then you can be a strong princess for Daddy."

"I daddy princess!"

"Yes, you are, and don't you ever forget that. Are you sure you don't want to watch something other than cartoons?"

"No!"

"Okay, yes, your majesty." She giggles. "One day, I will get you, but for now, I will allow you to be this way. After all, you are 3 years old. Just don't grow up so fast like your sister and brother did. Can you do that for Daddy?"

"Funny, Daddy, look!"

"It's okay, princess. I know you understand and hear everything I say to you."

As time goes by, Michael grows impatient. "Excuse me, Kayla?"

"Yes, Michael, what do you need?"

"I was just wondering if the results had come back yet."

"As a matter of fact, I was just about to tell you that. I already gave them to Dr. Lee, and she should see you soon."

"Well, that doesn't sound good."

"Don't worry, Michael. You know Jazmyn is in good hands here."

"I understand that, but you must understand. This is my princess."

"I can't pretend to understand how you feel, but just remember where you are. The doctor's specialty is what Jazmyn has, so she will explain everything to you soon."

"Can you give me a hint?"

"I am sorry, Michael. You know I can't do that. It is against policy. Even if I were able to tell you, she could explain what is going on with Jazmyn better than I can for you."

"Thank you for your honesty, Kayla."

"Any time, Michael."

He says a prayer in his head. *Lord, thank you for taking her pain away. Even though it was the treatment, it was you who invented it. Please give me the strength to handle any news that is to come. In your heavenly name, I pray, Lord. Amen.*

The nurse answers a call. "Yes, doctor. I will let him know immediately. Okay, doctor. Bye."

"Please tell me some good news, Kayla."

"The doctor would like to see you in her office, Michael. Do you remember where her office is located?"

"Yes. Unfortunately, I have been in there too many times. What about Jazmyn? I can't just leave her in here by herself."

"I will stay in here with her. Besides, I love spending time with her. Obviously, I wish it weren't under these circumstances."

"I hear you on that. Okay. Thank you, Kayla. Princess, Daddy will be back soon. Kayla is going to stay with you and watch cartoons with you. Okay?"

"'Kay."

"Keep being a strong girl for Daddy."

"Bye Daddy."

"Princess, remember you should never say bye. Say something like 'see you soon.'"

"Soon, Daddy."

Michael and Kayla laugh as Jazmyn giggles. "That is more like it, princess. I will be back."

Michael then leaves, and as he makes his way to the office, he has many thoughts racing through his head. *Oh Lord, let this be good news.* He knocks on the door. "Dr. Lee? It's Michael."

"The door is open, Michael."

He enters the room, not knowing what to expect.

"Hi, Michael. Please come in and have a seat. I already received an update, but I would like to hear it from you. How is Jazmyn doing?"

"She says she is feeling ill, but I know it is from her chemotherapy."

"I understand. Unfortunately, that side effect is common in cancer patients, especially children."

"To be honest, I, on the other hand, am extremely nervous."

"I understand, Michael. You know I don't beat around the bush, so I am going to just tell it to you like it is."

"That is what I admire about you, doctor, but please inform me what is going on with Jazmyn."

"As you know, Michael, Jazmyn is in stage II-A of her cancer, which means that the cancer, at the moment, is still in the area where it started and on one side of her body but not all of the visible tumor cannot be safely removed by surgery. Although treatments are somewhat helpful, I am afraid she is not responding well to her chemotherapy, and I am sorry to tell you that it's not enough to help her with her condition."

"Not enough for what?"

"I am sorry, Michael, but it does not appear to be good."

"Wait a minute! What exactly are you trying to tell me?!"

"I know this isn't easy for you to hear—"

"Well, yes, is it that obvious?"

"Please try to remain calm. I will explain it you in a way for you to understand it better. As you know, Jasmyn was diagnosed with neuroblastoma,
which is a rare but aggressive cancer. With the way that her condition is
progressing, I am afraid that treatments are not just doing enough for her."

"So, what do I do from here then?"

"As I said, her condition is rare and medicine has only gotten her this
far by a miracle. Most survivors of her condition suffer long-term effects,
and their health is poor at best. There are experimental treatments that I
can recommend for her. I, of course, will continue to treat and monitor
Jazmyn, but I do not want to give you false hope."

"I do not understand this, doctor! She is only three years old! Why is this
happening?!"

"Speaking from a medical prospective, I cannot give you an honest answer
on that."

"You must be wrong, doctor. There must be something we can do. God
would not allow this to happen to one of his children! No, I refuse to accept it!"

"Michael, I know you have your faith, and I admire that about you, but I
just don't have the answers you are searching for. I am only speaking to you
from a medical standpoint."

Michael puts his head down. "I just don't know what to do at this point,
doctor."

"Just be with her, Michael. At this point in her life, she needs family more
than anything else. I see the way you are with her. Continue to show her

as much love as possible. I am sorry, Michael. I will give you a moment to yourself. Please take all the time you need in my office." The doctor gets up and heads to the door.

"Doctor, there must be something we can do."

"There is, Michael. Just show her as much love as possible. Please do not hesitate to call me for anything you or Jazmyn needs. I must go make my rounds now. Please take care, Michael."

The doctor leaves, and Michael drops to his knees. "Lord, where are you?! Jazmyn is only 3 years old! She needs you now more than ever." Michael sobs. "I need you, Lord. Please. I will do anything you ask of me, Lord. Name it, it's done. Just tell me what to do. Please… Help us." Michael gets up, composes himself, and heads back to Jazmyn. "Hey princess. Feeling better?"

"Yup. Tired, Daddy."

"I know, princess. We should be able to get you home soon, and I will put you into bed to go night night."

"Yay," Jazmyn says groggily.

"How much time does she have left, Kayla?"

"Actually, she is just about done. How do you feel, Jazmyn?"

"Better."

"I am glad you said that, because you are all done. Let me take this out for you. Don't worry; it tickles coming out. There you are, Jazmyn. You were a very good girl today. I am sure your dad is very proud of you."

"I am, princess. You are my big girl."

"I big girl."

"Yes, you are, princess. Let's get your stuff and go home."

"'Kay, Daddy."

As Michael gathers Jazmyn's things into her bag, he thanks the nurse. "Thank you again, Kayla, for staying with her and for being so helpful today."

"Don't mention it, Michael. It was my pleasure. Bye, big girl."

"Bye," Jazmyn says as she wraps her hands around Michael's neck and puts her head into his chest.

"Bye, Michael. Take care."

"Goodbye, Kayla. Have a great day." Michael heads out into the waiting room.

"Daddy!" the children shout.

"Hey soldiers. Were you good for your aunts?"

"I was."

"Me too, Daddy."

"I believe you both. Yolanda, Aunt Ruthie, are you two ready to leave?"

"I am. These cuties know their way around this place. They were our tour guides."

"Unfortunately, that is true."

"Hey, Michael, you don't look all that well. What is wrong with you?"

"Aunt Ruthie, I will tell you and Yolanda later."

"Okay, Michael."

"I am going to say goodbye to Stephanie and then we can leave." He goes to the front desk. "I thank you so much, Stephanie, for getting her in as quickly as you did. You have no idea how much that meant to me."

"You are very welcome, Michael. I am just glad to see that she isn't in so much pain anymore. You guys take care, and Jazmyn, I want to see that beautiful smile of yours."

"Bye," Jazmyn says with a smile, waving.

"That is what I wanted to see."

"Thank you again, Stephanie. Have a great day."

"Thank you, Michael. Please do the same. Bye guys."

"Bye!" the children say, waving.

"Okay, soldiers, let's get this princess home so she can get some rest."

They exit the hospital, pile into the car, and head home.

"See, Jazzy? I told you that when you got you magic potion those meanies would go away."

"Yeah, Jazzy, and my special hug helped, too."

"That is sweet for both of you two to say. I know she appreciates your love for her."

"She keeps closing her eyes, Daddy. Is she tired?"

"Yes, sweetie, you know how sometimes your magic potions can make you guys sleepy."

"Oh, yeah we do."

"I know buddy. Believe me, I know."

Yolanda sees in Michael's eyes that something is troubling him. "Michael what happened at the hospital? Aunt Ruthie was right. There is something wrong with you."

"I can't discuss it in the car, especially with Annabelle and Gabriel here. I will inform you and Aunt Ruthie later, after I put them in bed."

"Okay, Michael, but you just don't look like yourself right now."

"I know, Yolanda. I just have so many thoughts racing through my mind right now. I just want to get home and let princess get some rest."

They arrive home and walk into the house.

"Soldiers, you can go on your electronic things, but please read something; don't just look at videos or play games on it."

"Okay, Daddy," the children say happily.

"Dinner will be ready shortly. I am going to put princess in her bed so she can get some rest."

"Night night, Jazzy. I love you," Gabriel says as he gives her a kiss.

"Goodnight, Jazzy. Love you," Annabelle says as she gives her a kiss.

"She loves you guys too. She is just tired. Yolanda, I will be back. I am going to make sure she is good and comfortable for bed and then I will start dinner."

"That's okay, Michael. I will make dinner."

"Are you sure?"

"Yes. It's no problem. What did you have in mind?"

"I was thinking spaghetti tonight. It's their favorite and since they behaved so well at Adventure Land today, I figured they should be rewarded for that. I just have one small request."

"What is it?"

"If you don't mind, please use the veggie pasta."

"Sure, Michael, I can do that."

"Thank you, Yolanda. You are the best. Aunt Ruthie, did you want to say goodnight to the princess?"

"Yes, I do. Goodnight, my sweet baby. You know I love you so much. You go get some rest now, so I can see that smile again." She kisses Jazmyn. "There you are, my baby girl."

"Okay, princess, time for night night." He takes her into her room.

"Tired, Daddy."

"I know, princess. That is why I am putting you in your bed. First, I need to put you in your pajamas… there you are. Let me just cover you up… and here is your goodnight bear. There, you are all set for bed now. I love you so much, my sweet princess. I know you don't really understand this now, but together with faith and love we will win."

"Love, you Daddy."

Michael smiles at her. "Do you want me to stay for a little bit?"

"Sleepy," she says, closing her eyes and clutching her bear.

"Okay, princess. I will let you rest up so you can be my strong princess again."

"'Kay." She falls asleep. Michael kisses her, and she can do nothing but stare at her.

"Lord, this your child. Why must she go through this?" He shuts the door and heads into the kitchen. "Wow, sis, dinner smells good!"

"What, are you surprised I can cook?"

"I apologize. I didn't mean for it to sound like that. I was just commenting on how good it smells."

"Okay, Michael, you are forgiven. Go ahead and bring the cuties over to the table. Dinner is ready."

"Will do. Okay, soldiers, come and get it!"

"Yes, I am starving!"

"I know you are, sweetie."

"What are we having, Daddy?"

"Well, buddy, since you two were so good today, Aunt Yolanda made spaghetti."

"Yes! Spaghetti!"

"That's right, buddy. Aunt Ruthie, did you do your log today?"

"I did, Michael."

"Okay, I was just checking. Everyone, please sit and I will get your plates."

"I've got it, Michael. Go ahead and sit."

"Thank you, sis."

Yolanda portions out the meals and serves everyone.

"Soldiers, what do you say?"

"Thank you, Aunt Yolanda!" they shout.

"You are very welcome, cuties. Enjoy."

"Wait a minute. First, we must thank the Lord for blessing us with this meal. Who wants to say grace?"

"I will, Daddy."

"Okay, sweetie. Whenever you are ready."

"Thank you, Lord, for this delicious meal you have blessed us with and for my family eating together except for Jazzy. Please heal her so we can all eat together again. Amen."

"Very good, sweetie. Thank you for that. Okay everyone, let's eat. So, Yolanda what did you guys do at Adventure Land?"

"We went everywhere. I know Gabriel is your son because he couldn't get enough of the sports room."

"That's my boy."

"And Annabelle, of course, was in the computer room with Aunt Ruthie."

"You were, sweetie?"

"Yeah, I was making videos in there."

"You know, you had your tablet."

"I know. I just wanted to stay in there because they have so many new cool programs in there."

Michael shaking his head. "I will never understand all this technology stuff."

Everyone laughs.

"I will say this, Michael, we felt like rock stars in there. Everyone knew who these cuties were."

"Unfortunately, that is true. I wish it weren't so, but the staff is great there."

"They are. They even gathered all the kids because some football player had stopped by."

"Really?! Who was it?"

"I don't know the name, but he must have been someone important because all the kids lit up when he came in."

"Yeah, Daddy, it was awesome!"

"You see what I mean, soldiers, by 'Adventure Land?' You never know what will happen there. I am glad to hear you guys were able to meet him, whoever it was."

"Michael, what about you? How was your visit?"

"Well, Aunt Ruthie, Jazmyn and I went into the room and she got her magic potion."

"Did the doctor take a look at her?"

"She did. She examined Jazzy and drew some blood."

"Then what happened?"

"Dr. Lee and I had what seemed to be a long conversation about what is going on with my princess."

"Okay. Don't leave us in suspense. Tell us what you two discussed."

"Aunt Ruthie, now is not the time. After I get them in bed, I will tell you and Yolanda what we had discussed."

"I will hold you to that, Michael."

"Soldiers, how is the food?"

"It's my favorite. Spaghetti! It's yummy!"

"I know it is your favorite, buddy."

"It's delicious, Aunt Yolanda."

"Well, thank you, Annabelle, and thank you, Gabriel, for your feedback. I am glad your cuties are enjoying it, Michael. Aunt Ruthie, are you enjoying the meal?"

"I am, Yolanda. It's delicious."

"Michael, what about you? How is it?"

"I agree with everyone here. It's real good. Thank you for cooking tonight."

"You're welcome, Michael."

"Soldiers, after you finish eating, line up for your medicines. Then I need you two to take your baths, and then it will be time for bed."

"Aw, man!"

"I know, buddy, but tomorrow, we go back to Adventure Land for your magic lasers. I need you to be well rested and strong to fight those meanies in you."

"Yeah, I am going to beat them up. Right, Daddy?"

"That's right, buddy. You are going to beat them meanies."

"What about me, Daddy?"

"Sweetie, I know you are strong as well. Remember: with hope, faith, and love, together we will defeat all those meanies."

"That's right, Daddy, because God is always protecting us."

"That's right, sweetie. He is. Okay, soldiers, it looks like you're finished eating. Are you both good and full?"

"I am, Daddy."

"Me too. My tummy is full."

"That's good, soldiers. Line up for your medicines."

"Okay," the children say, lining up.

"Here is yours, buddy."

"Thank you."

"You are welcome… and here is yours, sweetie."

"Thank you."

"You're welcome. Now, you both know what I am going to say."

"All done, Daddy. See?"

"Me too, Daddy."

"Good job, soldiers. I didn't even have to remind you guys to finish. I am proud of both of you. Okay, go ahead and get your baths out of the way."

"I'm first, sissy," Gabriel says as he runs off.

"Okay, buddy, but I don't want you to be stinky. Make sure you take a good bath."

"Okay!"

"Sweetie, go ahead and get your clothes ready and prepare for your bath."

"Okay, Daddy," Annabelle says. As she leaves, Michael begins to clean.

"So, Michael, are you going to tell us what happened today that is causing you so much pain? Or do we have to call the hospital and find out ourselves?"

"To be honest, Yolanda, I don't know what more I can do."

"What is troubling you, Michael?"

"Aunt Ruthie, Yolanda, I feel… well, I don't exactly know how I feel now."

"Just come out with it."

"It's just that I feel like my faith is being tested."

"How is your faith being tested? You know God has his reasons for everything that goes on within his creation, and he does not play games."

"I understand that, Aunt Ruthie. It's just that it clearly states in the Bible to ask and you shall receive. I ask and ask God to heal my children, but today I found out that Jazmyn's treatments aren't enough to help her anymore."

"What is that supposed to mean, Michael?!"

"It means, Yolanda, that her cancer is winning."

"Michael I am so sorry about everything you are going through with these babies and everything you went through when you lost Anna, but don't you dare lose your faith and trust in the Lord."

"I am trying so hard not to. It's just I don't know what more I can do. That is my princess and—"

"Daddy! I'm done!"

"Okay, buddy, I will be there in a minute! As I was saying, Yolanda, Aunt Ruthie, I just have a bad feeling about Annabelle and Gabriel's appointments."

"Don't start to think like that, Michael. Just don't. You do whatever you must do to help you get through this, and we are here to help you out any way that we can, but don't lose your faith and trust in the Lord like Aunt Ruthie just said."

"I know, and I am sorry for talking this way, but you both must realize that they are my children. They are God's children. I just don't understand why these things are happening."

"All you can do at this point, Michael, is pray."

"I know that Aunt Ruthie, and believe me, I pray often. Anyways, I am going to get them in bed and then I will be back out here to finish cleaning."

"I will finish this up, Michael. Go be with your children."

"We've got this, Michael. Go be with those babies of yours."

"Thank you both. I just wanted you two to know how much I appreciate everything you both do for us."

"As I told you before, Michael, we are family and that is what we do for each other—to always be here whenever you need us."

"I second that."

"Thank you again. I love you both so much. I am going to lie down with Jazmyn tonight. I will see you ladies in the morning. Goodnight."

"I love you too, Michael. Goodnight."

"Goodnight, Michael, and I will always love you like a son."

Michael smiles. "I am truly blessed that God gave me such a loving family such as yourselves." He gives each of them a hug and heads back to Gabriel. "Okay, buddy, here I am. I hope you are all clean."

"I am, Daddy. See? No stinky." Gabriel shows off his arms as Michael laughs.

"You are too much, buddy. Let's get you into bed. Are you ready for the goodnight prayer?"

"Yup."

"Okay let's say it together."

"As I lie down to sleep tonight, I pray to you, Lord, that you to keep my soul in your sight. I give you many thanks in the blessings you bring. Allow me to wake in the morning so that I may sing. In your name, I pray, Lord. Amen."

"Good job, buddy."

"Does Jesus hear me when I pray?"

"Of course he does, and as a matter of fact, I know that he loves you so much that he tells all of heaven to watch over you."

"Really, Daddy? All of heaven?"

"Yes, buddy. That is how much the Lord loves you."

"Wow!"

"Okay, buddy, let's see… you took your medicine, had a bath, you are tucked in, said your prayer… am I forgetting anything?"

"Daddy… monster check!"

Michael smiles. "You're right, buddy. I apologize. Let me see if any monsters are hiding. Nope, not in the closet."

"Bed!"

"Nope, not under the bed either. Looks like you are all set for night night. I love you my little buddy. Goodnight."

"Goodnight, Daddy. Love you too."

Michael shuts the door halfway and goes to Annabelle's room. "Okay, sweetie. Are you ready for bed?"

"Yeah, I am ready."

"That's my girl. I know you're growing up on me, and soon you won't need me to tuck you in."

"I will always be your little girl though."

He smiles at her.

"Yes, you are sweetie."

"Is Jazzy going to be okay, Daddy?"

"Of course, Annabelle. Why do you ask?"

"Well I'm a big girl now, and I know when something is wrong with you. Today, you looked so sad."

"I am sorry about that sweetie, but yes, she will be okay. All of you will. Are you ready for your bedtime prayer?"

"I am. I would like to say one for Jazzy if that is okay."

"Yes, sweetie, that is always okay, and you never need to ask permission to say a prayer for your family. A prayer is an open line between you and heaven."

"Okay, Daddy. Dear Lord, please heal Jazzy so she will feel better. I want her to grow up to be a big girl like me. Please heal Bubby and me so we can grow up big and strong like Daddy. Thank you for everything you bless us with. In your name, I pray, Lord. Amen. Was that good, Daddy?"

Michael, holding back his tears, softly tells her, "That was very good, sweetie. I love you so much. Goodnight."

"Goodnight, Daddy. I love you so much too."

He closes the door and goes to lie down with Jazmyn, whispering to her, "Princess, you are my soldier and God's child. Please fight for me. I love you so much, and I know they do in heaven as well, but I need you to be strong for me. I will never give up on you, so please don't give up the fight. I love you, princess." With tears in his eyes he falls asleep.

Chapter 7

"Daddy, Daddy, wake up!"

"I'm up, princess. I'm up."

"You went night night with me."

"I did. I see you are feeling better today."

"Yup."

"That is good. Where is my cheek?"

"Here."

"Let me get that little cheek."

As she giggles, he kisses her on the cheek. "Okay, princess, let's go get breakfast started before your brother and sister come out."

"'Kay."

They go into the kitchen and Michael starts breakfast.

"Daddy. Toons!"

"Princess, I know you love your cartoons, but there are some educational shows I want you to watch. They teach you numbers and letters. I am sure you will like them. It makes learning fun. Plus, you get to learn things so you can be a big girl."

"I big girl."

"That you are, but I need you to start learning your numbers and letters so when you are ready to go to school, you will be all caught up."

"'Kay."

"Besides, it will be fun. Here, I will show you. Let me find one that you will like… there you are, princess. It even has the animals that you love so much."

"Daddy look. Piggy."

"Very good, princess. Now please sit here in your chair and learn something while Daddy finishes cooking. Okay?"

"'Kay."

Michael puts Jazmyn in her chair and proceeds to finish cooking. As usual, Annabelle and Gabriel come running out.

"Daddy!"

"Good morning, soldiers. Gabriel, I love seeing you two every morning but what am I going to ask you both?"

"Aw man!"

Michael smiles at Gabriel. "Buddy, do me a favor. From now on, before you come running out, ask yourself this: what is Daddy going to ask me? Can you do that from now on?"

"Yes, sir."

"Daddy isn't trying to be mean, buddy. Gabriel, I will explain it better to both of you. I love you all so much that I want you all to do things on your own. There is going to be a point in your lives that I won't be there to annoy you with those types of questions and to remind you about your medicines, baths, and prayers."

"Where are you going, Daddy?" Annabelle asks with a concerned look on her face.

"I am never going to leave you guys. I will always be with you all. The point that I am trying to make is that, when you get older and live in your own houses, I won't be there to remind you guys of normal activities."

"But I like it here, Daddy."

"Me too. I don't want to go nowhere else."

Michael smiles. "I love you soldiers so much, and you guys are always welcome to stay if you want. As I explained it to you all, family is always going to be here whenever you need us. I am just speaking in the sense that when you go to college and start careers, there is going to be a time when you decide that you will want to move into your own places and live somewhere other than here."

"I'm never leaving, Daddy."

"Me neither. I love it here."

Michael smiles again. "This will always be your home, soldiers, and if or when the time comes in the point of your lives, you will then understand what I am trying to say. You can go ahead and brush your teeth, buddy."

"Okay." He runs off.

"I always brush my teeth, Daddy."

"I know you do, sweetie. You know what else I am going to ask."

"I know and I have to be honest my chest has been weird again."

"How so?"

"It just feels like someone is squeezing it again. It doesn't really hurt. It just feels weird. It only lasts about five-teen or so minutes."

"I called your doctor the last time you told me you felt this way and she explained to me that it was called angina."

"What is that?"

"It's when you do physical exertion."

"Huh?"

"It means sweetie that when you do too much running or things like that, your heart is doing too much. Your heart muscle doesn't get enough oxygen, and that is why you are feeling like someone is squeezing your chest. She said that there are two types—stable and unstable."

"What do I have then?"

"You have stable, which is everything I just described."

"What is the other?"

"Unstable is a more concerning symptom because that is a chest pain that happens without you doing any activities. That is why I am constantly asking you if you are feeling well. You must be careful when you do things. You don't want to overwork your body, especially your heart. So, please, by all means, tell me when you have these types of pain. Even though I explained it to you casually, it is still a concern. So, please never brush off anything you are feeling."

Gabriel comes back out. "All clean, Daddy. See?"

"Good job, buddy. I was just explaining to your sister about something, so I want both of you two to listen to me. Those meanies in you guys are tough and sneaky in some of the things they are doing to you guys. I know you soldiers tell me all the time that you are okay, but never leave even the littlest of things out. However you are feeling, I want to know immediately so that I can ask your doctors about what you soldiers are going through. You soldiers are tough and have faith, but we also need knowledge."

"What's that, Daddy?"

"Buddy, knowledge means to have information."

"You tell us all we need is hope, faith, and love to help us defeat the meanies."

"Annabelle, that is very true, and with those traits, you soldiers will defeat anything that tries to attack you, but we also need knowledge. Your doctors and I need to know as much information as possible about your conditions and meanies to help you soldiers fight them. So, when I ask you soldiers all the time how you are feeling, it's not because I ask just to ask. It is because I need as much information as possible to help the doctors so I understand what exactly is causing you soldiers to go through with anything that you are going through.

"I know I sound like a broken record all the time, but you soldiers must understand how much I care for you all. I don't care what time it is, where we are, or what we are doing. If you two sense that something is wrong, don't ever be afraid to tell me. Your doctors and I are not mind-readers. Yes, your doctors are highly trained and very good at their jobs, but they can only help you with what they see with your tests. I, on the other hand, didn't go to school to learn about your meanies. I only know from what you soldiers and the doctors tell me. So, we all are in this together. I need to know everything possible. That is why I ask you soldiers those questions all the time. It is so that I can tell the doctors.

"For example, Annabelle, you did very good telling me about your chest feeling like someone is squeezing it because had you not told me that. I wouldn't had been able to ask your doctor what was causing it and as she explained to me it was a normal symptom from your condition. I say normal loosely because nothing is normal with your meanies. So, please even if you two think it's nothing to worry about, tell me and I will then ask your doctors. With even the littlest information they get from you soldiers, they can better treat the meanies."

"Like when Jazzy was crying yesterday, Daddy?"

"Yes, sweetie, but she is only 3 years old, so that was her way of telling me that something was wrong. You two, on the other hand, are much older, and, as I said before, I cannot read your minds. Gabriel, I will use you as an example. I know that because today is the day you get your magic lasers, your stomach is hurting. Am I correct?"

"Yeah, but I wanted you to think I am a strong big boy like you."

Michael smiles. "Buddy, I know you are very strong but if your doctors had not told me that you soldiers will feel some discomfort on days of your magic potions, I would just think that you soldiers were okay. Just by looking at you buddy and the way you are happy, I would just continue to think that you were fine, but knowing what I know, I know that is not the case."

"My tummy does hurt, Daddy."

"I know it does, buddy, but when you feel that way or have any feeling that you aren't feeling all that well, then tell me. Am I understood? Did I make myself clear? Or do you want me to explain it better for you two?"

"No, I understand everything you are saying, Daddy."

"Me too, Daddy."

"That's good to hear, soldiers. I just wanted to let you guys in on why I ask you two so many questions. Come here, soldiers." Michael hugs them both.

"I love hugs from you, Daddy."

"I know you do, buddy."

"I do too, bubby."

"I know you do, sweetie. I will finish getting breakfast out now. While I do this, I want you two to go read something, and I don't care if it's on your electronic things. All I care is if both of you read something."

"Okay." Gabriel runs off.

"I always read, Daddy."

"I know you do, sweetie."

"Did you—"

"Yes, I already logged you guys into those things. Annabelle, please remember that you must take it easy."

"Okay, I will." She goes into the living room at the same moment that Yolanda comes out.

"Good morning, cuties."

"Good morning, Aunt Yolanda!" Annabelle and Gabriel shout.

"Hi Jazzy. I see you are feeling better."

Jazmyn giggles. "Yeah."

"That's good to hear, cutie. Good morning, Michael. Breakfast sure does look good today."

"Thank you, Yolanda, and good morning to you as well."

"So, where did you sleep last night?"

"I feel asleep in princess' bed next to her."

"You actually slept? After what you told us, I didn't know if you were going to sleep or not. Especially with the way you looked."

"Admittingly, so many thoughts were racing through my head, but in the end, I just turned to my faith as you and Aunt Ruthie suggested."

"That's good, Michael."

"Besides, I sort of had a pep talk with Jazmyn as she lay there in her bed."

"You two talked?"

"No, she was sleeping. I just whispered words of encouragement to her."

"Well good. As I said last night, you do what you must do to get you through everything."

"Unfortunately, we are not out of the woods yet. Gabriel goes in for his treatment today, and as usual, his stomach is hurting. We also get the results back to confirm what Doctor Smith has a strong suspicion is causing Gabriel's pain."

"I hope it's not DSRCT, Michael."

"I pray that isn't the case either, but to be honest with you, if it is DSRCT then at least his doctor was smart enough to figure it out. That is why he had surgery awhile back, and that is why he goes in for..." Michael whispers to Yolanda, "...radiation therapy."

"I don't understand something about that, Michael. If he only suspected that that was what's causing Gabriel's pain, then why did he give him surgery and why are they giving him that type of treatment based solely on suspicion?"

"I didn't understand that either, but as you know, he was suffering from many symptoms like having pain in the stomach, cramping, nausea, and constipation. I took him to the only place I trusted—Adventure Land."

"Why didn't you take him to a regular hospital?"

"Because since Annabelle and Jazmyn go there, I figured that it was the one place that could properly evaluate him. Don't get me wrong, there are a lot of good hospitals out there, but unfortunately, since I knew the staff so well at Adventure Land, I figured that he was in the best of hands there. I was right for taking him there because they immediately identified the issue he was having. So we were referred to Dr. Smith who is a specialist at Adventure Land."

"I know I don't know that much about all this medical stuff, but it just seems odd to me that a doctor of his stature would operate on a patient and give him... well, magic lasers without first knowing exactly what was wrong with the patient."

"That's the thing. Dr. Smith is a specialist and a very good doctor at that. He has been practicing medicine for over 20 years, and he immediately knew what was causing Gabriel's pain. He at first thought it was just cancer, and no, I am not saying that like it is just some kind of condition. Cancer is very serious, but Dr. Smith explained to me there are so many cancers out there, and they all are very tricky. Sometimes the doctors know which cancer a patient suffers from immediately, and other times what they first think is one cancer turns out to be another—just like in Gabriel's case.

"He thought it was just a tumor but operated on Gabriel and found out it that was something else after he couldn't safely remove it. That is why Gabriel had all those tests done last week, and now unfortunately, today, we find out if its DSRCT or not. I trust all the staff at Adventure Land, and I trust a doctor who has been in practice for over 20 years. So when he says that that is what Gabriel is suffering from, then I will take all the advice and treatments he recommends. I know it is hard to comprehend why a doctor will treat a patient based on suspicion, but I have read about DSRCT, and even Dr. Smith agrees that with all the information, this is the road we are at.

"Trust me, Yolanda, I pray that he doesn't have it, but I also pray to the Lord that he brought us Dr. Smith because if he does have DSRCT, then at least Gabriel has a head start on fighting it. What I am most afraid of is if that is by the time it gets diagnosed, it will already have spread. I can only take comfort in the fact that Dr. Smith is already treating Gabriel as if that is what he has because he will be in for one heck of a fight."

"Wow, Michael. It must be tough not knowing. I can't even pretend what I would do if I were in your shoes, but I agree that at least now if he does have that then the doctor already is treating him."

"Trust me, Yolanda. It's not going to be pretty after my conversation with the doctor today. Do you see why I said yesterday that I have a bad feeling about Gabriel and Annabelle's appointments?"

"I do, Michael. I do, and I don't blame you one bit for thinking the way you do. Just remember what Aunt Ruthie and I said last night—whatever happens today and tomorrow, do not lose your faith and trust in the Lord. We are also here for you and those cuties."

"I appreciate that, Yolanda. I really do. Anyways, where is Aunt Ruthie? Breakfast is done. She is usually out here by now."

"I don't know. I will go check on her." Aunt Ruthie walks out. "Oh, I found her, Michael. Here she is."

Michael and Yolanda both laugh.

"Oh, ha-ha, you two."

"Good morning, Aunt Ruthie."

"Good morning, Yolanda. Good morning Michael."

"You know I love seeing that beautiful face in the morning, Aunt Ruthie. What took you so long?"

"I had to log my readings."

"How are they?"

"The usual. High blood pressure. Normal sugar levels."

"Well, we must do something to bring that pressure down, Aunt Ruthie."

"Yeah, yeah. You sound just like my doctor. Breakfast looks good. What are we having?"

"Don't try to change the subject." She smiles.

"Since Gabriel goes in for his magic lasers today, I made his favorite: pancakes, eggs, and bacon."

"Can he have all that grease and starch?"

"I will let you both in on a secret." He whispers to Yolanda and Aunt Ruthie, "It's whole wheat cakes, organic eggs, and turkey bacon."

"Is that why they look so different?"

"Yes, but they love it. And as Anna did to me, what they don't know won't hurt them. If they eat, then I am okay with cooking stuff like this."

"You are a good father, Michael."

"Thank you, Aunt Ruthie. I try to be. You ladies can sit; I will serve everyone. Okay, soldiers, come and get it!"

"Yes! Finally!"

"I heard that, sweetie."

"Daddy, is that what I think it is?"

"It is buddy, and I even made it into a smiley face for you and Jazzy."

"Yes!"

"Okay everyone, please have a seat at the table. Princess, here is your smiley face."

"Yay!" she says with excitement as Michael smiles.

"Eat up princess, and don't just admire it like last time."

"'Kay."

"Okay, here you all are." He serves everyone. "Okay. As we always should do, we must thank the Lord for this meal. Any volunteers?"

"I will, Michael."

"Okay, Yolanda. We are ready when you are."

"Everyone, please bow your heads and put your hands together."

They all do so.

"Dear Lord, we are most grateful for this meal and the many things that you provide for us. We also are very thankful that we all are eating together as one family. Please guide us through our day as some of us will need you more than others. We always are thankful for providing for us every day with the strength you bless us with to live our lives. In your heavenly name, Jesus, we pray. Amen."

They all say together, "Amen."

"Thank you, Yolanda. That meant a lot. Okay everyone, let's eat."

"Yeah!" Gabriel says happily.

"Buddy, I need you to finish all your meal. I need you big and strong for your magic lasers today so you can fight those meanies."

"Oh, I am, Daddy. Imma eat it all up, then I'm going to beat up those meanies. Imma go *boom*! And *bam*! And those meanies are going to run! Right, Daddy?"

Everyone laughs.

"That is right, buddy."

"And tomorrow when I get my magic potion, I'm going to beat up the meanies too. Right, Daddy?"

"That's right, sweetie, you will."

"This is delicious, Michael."

"I agree with Yolanda."

"Well, thank you both, ladies. I am glad that my family enjoys my cooking."

"Daddy… can I ask you a question?"

"Of course, sweetie. What is it?"

"You tell us all the time about family and talk to us how important it is to us…but what is the definition of family?"

"Wow, sweetie, I didn't expect that, but…" Everyone looks at Michael and listens. "Family is true happiness—that is the cornerstone to any foundation in life. Most people get confused about what family is and what it's supposed to be."

"Like how, Daddy?"

"Well, sweetie, unfortunately, there are some in families that only care about what each other has. Some just care about material possessions such as money, cars, and who has the biggest house. Some see families as a bank and only call each other for one reason—to see how much they can get from them. Some family members take advantage of each other just to see how much they can get out of one another. Just because they are related, they think that they are intitled to do so, but that isn't family. That is not what God intended family to be. You see, your grandma taught your aunt and me that just because you share genes with someone, that doesn't automatically make you family."

"It doesn't?"

"No, buddy, it does not. People often forget that we all share blood with one another. That is one thing most people forget. Is the fact that God created all of us with the same blood going through our veins. It doesn't matter what race, religion, or nationality we are. We all bleed the same blood. He knew his reasons when he created us that way, and I have a theory why."

"Why Daddy?"

"You see, buddy, true family is someone that you can talk to and laugh and cry with. Family is someone that God has put in your life to help guide you through life. True family is someone that will ask you 'How I can help guide you through your troubles?' Someone who is there with you through not only the good times in your life but the bad times as well. As I told you guys before, family will always be there when you need them.

"The best way you will know when you are in the presence of family is by their actions. There is an old saying about giving someone the shirt off their back, and what that means is that they will do whatever they can for you. Real family will say things such as 'If you are hungry, I will feed you. If you are tired, I will give you a place to rest. If you need clothes, I will provide them for you.' As it says in the Bible, do onto others as you would want done unto you.

"You see soldiers, we were blessed with such a wonderful family because of aunt Yolanda and aunt Ruthie coming to live with us. It's funny that they think we took them in. Yes, this may be the home God blessed us with, but it was they who took us in. Aunt Yolanda needed a place to stay, and God blessed us with such a big home that we had a room for her. She cleans, cooks, looks after you guys, and is always around when I need her. Then there is Aunt Ruthie. She was lost in life, and unfortunately after her husband, my uncle, went home to be in heaven, she didn't know where to turn to."

"Like Mommy did, Daddy?"

"Yes, sweetie. You see, soldiers, there are some so-called family members out there that just care about themselves and forget about everyone else out in the world, but we are fortunate to have Aunt Yolanda and Aunt Ruthie in our lives living here with us. The reason why I said they took us in is because they bring so much love to us and that is something that we needed more than anything. They are what completes us as a family. As I said to you, some people only see material things and they seem to forget the most valuable thing in this world, the thing you can't buy with money.

It's so priceless that you can have all the money in the world, but you still wouldn't be able to purchase it. Can you soldiers think what that is?"

"Love!" the children shout.

"That is right, soldiers. Love and those traits that I explained to you all. That right there is the definition of true family."

"Wow… like we are, Daddy?"

"That is right, buddy. Because all of us love and care for one another, we are a perfect example of a family."

"Thanks for telling us that, Daddy."

"You're welcome, sweetie. Okay. Looks like you soldiers are finished with your meals. Is everyone good and full? Gabriel, I am looking at you, buddy."

"Yup, I'm all done."

"I'm full too, Daddy."

"Okay, soldiers, line up for medicine time."

"Okay. Me first, sissy."

"Buddy, remember what I said about ladies first?"

"Oh, I'm sorry, sissy."

"It's okay bubby today you go in for magic lasers, and I know your tummy is hurting. You can go first."

Michael smiles. "Okay, here is yours, buddy."

"Thank you."

"You're welcome. And here is your cup, sweetie."

"Thank you, Daddy."

"You're welcome. Princess, here are yours—drink them with your juice."

"'Kay."

"All gone, Daddy."

"Mine too, Daddy."

"Good job, soldiers. Now please go get dressed and get ready to leave for Adventure Land."

"Yay! Adventure Land!" the children shout as they leave.

"Gone."

"Good job, princess. Daddy must clean up and then we will go get dressed."

"Don't bother, Michael. I will take care of it."

"No, Yolanda, I can't allow you to clean this up. Besides, you are always very helpful around here, and although I am very appreciative of your generosity, I made this mess, and it is my responsibility to clean it up."

"After what you just said, Michael, it is the least I can do for you."

"I didn't say that to get you two to do more around here. I was just explaining what I thought family meant to me. That is all I meant by it."

"Michael, you must understand something, and, Aunt Ruthie, you can agree or disagree with me on this, but when you first took us in, we didn't know what to expect. You were a newly widowed father with three very ill children, but the way you all present yourselves as a family and the way you all accepted Aunt Ruthie and me with open arms meant a lot to us. You and those cuties have so much love that it's contagious. Every day I just sit here and admire the way you are with your children. You make sure they read often, you make sure they know who the Lord is—the way you all love each other and the way you speak to them... it's as if you don't see their illnesses. You just see your children, and that is very admirable.

"You do so many things that I myself wouldn't know where to begin with when I wake up in the morning. That is not the case with you. You plan out your schedule and follow it to every detail. With all that you do for those cuties, Aunt Ruthie, and me, it is the very least that I can do for you = to clean up around here.

"You are right about the definition of family, and I was very touched by what you just told us. To be honest I am always moved by anything you tell those cuties. Be it about life or whatever you are talking about at that moment, I make sure to be close so I can listen to your speech. I'm not speaking for anyone else, but I am so proud of you and I know in heaven they all feel the same up there about what you are doing down here on Earth."

"Michael there is nothing to be said after what Yolanda just said. I agree with her 100 percent. I will say this, though, I know for a fact that they are smiling in heaven at the way you are raising those babies and the way you treat everyone as if they are your family. Anyone around you for even just a few minutes can sense that."

At that moment, Michael is filled with so many emotions. "Thank you both for that. It means a lot, not only to me but to my soldiers, that both of you are here with us. God has truly blessed us."

"Daddy, pretty."

"I know, princess. I know Daddy must get you ready. As a matter of fact, so do I."

"Go get yourself and those cuties ready, Michael."

"Okay. Thank you again, Yolanda. Both of you are coming right?"

"Of course we are. Why do you think Aunt Ruthie and I are dressed?"

"We are always where you and those babies need us, Michael."

"I love you ladies so much."

"We love you too, Michael."

"You must hurry because you know those cuties are going to hound you on not being ready."

"Okay, okay, I am going now. Let's go, princess. Time to get ready."

"Yay!"

Michael then takes Jazmyn to get dressed.

"Daddy! We have to go. My tummy hurts!"

Michael rushes to the door where everyone is waiting. "I'm sorry, buddy. Sorry everyone. I have my keys... wait, where are their bags?"

"I grabbed them, Michael, while you were getting ready. I put them in the car."

"Thank you, Yolanda. I packed them last night, so I think we are set to leave now. Let me just set the alarm and lock the door." He does so. "Okay everyone, please get in the car."

They all pile in the car.

"Everyone buckled in?"

"Yeah!" the children shout.

"So am I, Michael."

"Okay, sis, looks like you are too. Okay, let's go to Adventure Land."

"Yay!" the children shout.

They then get on the road and head to the hospital.

"Hey buddy, how are you feeling back there?"

"My tummy hurts, Daddy."

"I know it does, buddy, but we are almost there."

"Okay."

"Don't worry, bubby. You will feel all better soon."

They arrive at the hospital and take the elevator to the children's floor.

"Okay, buddy, we are here."

"Good, because I need to beat up these meanies—they are hurting me."

"Stay strong, buddy. Remember: you are a soldier."

"Okay."

"Yolanda, they are most likely to take him back right away since it's so close to his appointment. You already have the girls' bags. Their medicines are in each of their bags. Don't worry—they are counted out and labeled on the little baggies. Here is my card so they can eat something to take their afternoon meds. It is almost time for them to take them, and as always, just follow them to wherever they want to go. Please make sure they eat before taking their meds, okay?"

"I've got it, Michael. Good luck, cutie."

"Thank you, Aunt Yolanda."

All the girls leave. Michael and Gabriel go to the check-in desk. "Hi, Stephanie. I have the urge to say it's nice to see you again, but you know how it is under these circumstances."

"I know, Michael. I wish we could stop meeting like this as well. How are you two doing today?"

"I am good. It's my little buddy here who needs his magic lasers. The meanies are hurting him."

"Aw handsome, I am sorry to hear that. But we are going to fix that right up for you. Are you ready for your magic lasers, handsome?"

"Yeah I am, because Imma beat them meanies up! Right, Daddy?"

"Yes, you are, buddy."

Stephanie smiles. "That's good to hear. And guess what?"

"What?"

"Your girlfriend, Pamela, is here, and she will take you back there for your magic lasers. What do you think about that?"

Gabriel blushes as Michael smiles.

"Don't mind him; he calls her his girlfriend all the time."

"Daddy…" Gabriel says embarrassed.

"Do you know how long it will be until he goes back there?"

"She should be out any minute now. I called her as soon as I saw you guys."

"Thank you so much, Stephanie."

"Michael, you know it's no problem. We love your children. I wish it were under different circumstances, but that's neither here nor there. We are always here to help and happy to do so."

"I appreciate that, Stephanie."

"I wish I didn't have to say this but anytime, Michael."

"Trust me, Stephanie, I know."

The nurse comes out. "I heard my little boyfriend was out here."

Gabriel hides behind Michael.

"Now, where could he be hiding? There you are! Are you ready for your magic lasers so you can feel better?"

"Yup!"

"Okay, my little man, it's time to get you set up."

"Okay!"

"Hi Pamela. Let's go, buddy! It's time to beat up those meanies."

They go back into the treatment room.

"Hi Michael. How is he feeling today?"

"The usual. He looks and sounds happy, but I know he is hurting."

"Don't worry, we will fix that for him shortly."

"Is this going to hurt, Daddy?"

"No, buddy, remember we already went through the simulation process where your treatment team knows exactly where to treat you. They even made a special place for you to lie so you will be comfortable."

"Oh yeah."

"Pamela, can I talk to you for a minute?"

"Sure."

They move away from Gabriel.

"Doctor Smith already tried to explain why Gabriel needs this therapy, but why was it green lit if he wasn't certain it's DSRCT?"

"I understand your concern. After Doctor Smith performed surgery to try to remove the tumor, he noticed some irregularities. So, after the tests and the biopsy were performed, he had a physical and the treatment team reviewed Gabriel's medical history. Together they concluded that this was the best treatment. His treatment team sort of did their maps for the position of each treatment and the exact location of where the radiation will be given. That is why Dr. Smith, as you know, is an excellent oncologist. He determined his treatment plan and what machines to use. Don't worry. Gabriel will be just fine. Didn't Dr. Smith explain all of this to you?"

"He did, but I had a conversation with my sister, and she made a lot of sense asking why a doctor would give this type of treatment solely based on suspicion. Unless—wait…he does have DSRCT, doesn't he?"

"I really think you need to speak with Dr. Smith immediately, because this type of treatment isn't given out like it is aspirin. No doctor, at least one with a license, would ever recommend radiation therapy to just anyone unless they knew the exact cause for the treatment. Are you sure he didn't go over this with you? Because we can't treat a child without the parents signing off on it."

"He did, and we had several discussions about what I thought was just a suspicion of being DSRCT. So yes, I agreed to go along with this treatment. I'm not just going to put my son through this kind of treatment without knowing all the facts, but he did have a long discussion with me. All he talked about was how Gabriel is suffering from DSRCT, but I didn't realize he was certain. At least now that I think about it… I didn't want to believe it was true. You know me by now, Pamela. I am not some dumb father who just goes along with the flow without knowing facts first, because as you said it's not just an everyday treatment. I honestly just assumed the treatment team was just targeting the cancer and that was why Dr. Smith recommended this for him."

"Michael, I know you seemed shocked right now, but did you ever wonder why an oncologist with over 20 years of experience would recommend this type of treatment on just a suspicion?"

"No that's the thing I was under the impression that this was normal for cancer."

"Michael, it is, but what do you think DSRCT is?"

"From what I read, it's very serious."

"That's right; it is, and there is no doctor out there that will just say 'let's just put my patient under radiation therapy without knowing why.' He had to have told you all this so you would understand because if you didn't know, why would you have agreed to this based on a doctor's suspicion?"

"To be honest, I think—no, I know—he did in fact tell me, but because of the severity of the situation, I wanted to believe in my heart that Gabriel didn't have DSRCT. With Annabelle and Jazmyn already diagnosed with rare cancers," Michael put his head down, "I just didn't want to believe that

Gabriel had one as well. I hate myself for saying this, but I was just hoping it was only a normal cancer."

"Michael, cancer isn't normal. No matter what type of cancer a patient has, none of it is normal. I just can't believe he wouldn't have explained all this to you because that does not sound like him to do that, and it's definitely not what we would allow an oncologist to do—to just recommend something like this type of treatment."

"No, he did. It's just when we had discussed it, I heard 'suspicious' and my mind just went into overdrive and all I could get out of the conversation was that word. 'Suspicious.' So, I know deep inside I was in denial like I was when my girls were diagnosed. The same thing happened with them. I had to hear about their diagnoses several times and my then wife sat me down and explained it to me. Now that she isn't here anymore, I just didn't want to believe the doctor was right all along."

"Michael, we can stop now so that you can speak with Dr. Smith, because as I said, the parents have to sign off on all treatments, and I know you wouldn't have signed off on it without knowing for sure."

"No, he really needs this. I knew all along. I just didn't want to believe it was true. I knew he had a cancer, but I didn't want to believe it was a rare one like my girls'. I will go talk to him while Gabriel is in here."

"Are you sure? His treatment team is all here and ready to begin, but we will pull the plug. All I need is your say-so."

"No, please continue. I will go have a talk with Dr. Smith."

"Okay, Michael. We are going to begin. Do you remember where his office is located?"

"Unfortunately, I do."

"I will call ahead of time so that he will be expecting you. I believe that he is already expecting you to discuss some other matters."

"To be honest, in my mind it was to discuss what the tests results were, but as I think about it, he already has. How can I be so irresponsible about this?"

"Michael, you are dealing with enough already with your girls' conditions. Trust me, I see this a lot in parents who hear a diagnosis. It happens more often than you think. You are not alone."

"Pamela, that is what scares me. Isn't there enough in this world to deal with? Now children left and right have these types of illnesses and some don't even get to see their next birthday."

"I know you turned this down before, but there are support groups that meet here at the hospital and many more outside of the hospital, as well. There are also support groups online."

"I know, Pamela, and I appreciate what you are trying to do, but I will stay with my faith. Thank you. I will be leaving now."

"Okay, Michael. Just think about it."

"I will. Thank you. So when does he begin?"

"The team already prepped Gabriel while we were talking. He is set for his treatment."

"Okay, thank you, Pamela. Hey, buddy, look at you. Who is my big strong soldier who is going to fight the meanies today?"

"I am!"

"That's right, buddy, you are."

"Are you going to stay with me, Daddy?"

"I can't, buddy. The magic lasers only work for you, so I can't be here in the room with you. But as soon as you're done, I will be waiting right outside for you."

"Okay, Daddy."

"Give me one of your special hugs, buddy."

"Okay, I will give you a big special one!"

They both hug each other.

"Thank you, buddy, I needed that. Be good, and remember, what are you?"

"I'm a soldier!"

"That's right, buddy, you are. I will see you soon, buddy."

"Okay Daddy!"

Michael leaves the treatment room with a worried expression on his face and then walks down to the doctor's office and knocks on the door. "Hello, Dr. Smith, it's Michael."

"Yes, come in, Michael."

He enters the office.

"Please have a seat."

"I will be honest. I sat in Jazmyn's doctor's office yesterday, and she and I did not have a pleasant conversation."

"I understand what must be going through your head at the moment."

"I don't think you do, doctor, but it finally hit me in Gabriel's treatment room what is going on with him."

"Let's talk about that for a minute."

"I only have 30 minutes until Gabriel is finished."

"I received a strange call from the nurse that you were in shock about his diagnosis."

"I was in shock, and to be honest, I still am."

"As you know from our many conversations, what Gabriel has in fact is DSRCT."

"I know that now, doctor. It's just that every time we spoke, you said he had cancer and not that cancer is just something to play with words on, but I honestly didn't comprehend what you were telling me. I just didn't want to believe you. I do not understand how we arrived at this point. I heard everything you were saying to me, and I understood you, but something in me wanted to believe that you were wrong.

"Please don't think differently about me because of this, but I understand one child having cancer…but all three? And to make it worse, all three have rare cancers. It just doesn't add up. What are the odds of that happening? How can that possibly be? Anna and I do not have these diseases, so how did this happen to our children?"

"By now you know me, and I will never say anything disrespectful to you because I sympathize with everything that you are going through with your children. But I have to be blunt with you. I will give you some cold hard facts. To start, the odds of a child developing cancer by the age of 19 are 1 in 330, and you have three children with cancer, so you can do the math on that. I am sorry to say that it is quite an anomaly. To answer your question about family history, there are many cases in which cancer is caused by an abnormal gene that is passed down through generations. That is why your other children's doctors requested your family's history. I believe that to be the factor in Gabriel's case. I believe he inherited not the cancer itself but the abnormal gene that lead to the cancer. That brings me to why I asked you here today."

"I may not be ready to hear this, but I am listening."

"As you know by now, DSRCT is very rare. When we had operated on Gabriel to try to remove at least 90 percent of the tumor, unfortunately I was too late."

"Too late for what exactly?"

"It had metastasized. By the time we were able to diagnose Gabriel with DSRCT, it had already spread to other parts of the body."

"So, help me understand this, doctor."

"At first, I had thought that he had a stationary tumor and that I could safely remove it. After we operated, I found that not to be the case. That is why I did the biopsy. When I knew it was DSRCT, you and I had a very long discussion about it."

"I remember, doctor, but please tell me what you are trying to say."

"What I am trying to tell you, Michael, and please listen to me very carefully on this, is that DSRCT is so rare that there are no standard ways of treating it. Because so few people have DSRCT, only a small amount of information on treatment results are available. The only treatment methods that have been used on patients with DSRCT are surgery, chemotherapy, and radiation therapy. After extensive research and advice from my colleagues, I found that radiation therapy was the best method possible for Gabriel. That is why he is in there now getting treatment. I know you know this, because we had discussed this already, and you agreed with me on it."

"Dr. Smith, I agreed on his treatment because I trust this hospital and you because you are a specialist in your field. That's why I went with your judgment. Please tell me it's not true what they say about this cancer."

"Unfortunately, Michael, the little information we do have on this type of cancer tells us that it's true. Currently DSRCT has a 15 percent five-year survival rate. Researchers are looking for treatments that will improve those odds, but I must be honest with you; from where we are at now with Gabriel, it won't help. I am sorry to tell you this, Michael, but medically speaking, it doesn't appear to look good for Gabriel."

"Forgive me, Dr. Smith, but what is it with you doctors and saying 'medically speaking' all the time? Yesterday, Dr. Lee told me that she could only speak from a medical standpoint, and I know that Dr. Gomez will say the same thing tomorrow. I know it's coming, Dr. Smith, because bad news happens in threes. It's not just a myth—I know this to be a fact because just look at my children, doctor! Three of them get diagnosed with not only cancer but with rare cancers! Yesterday I heard that Jazmyn's treatments aren't enough to help her, and today you are telling me that the medical field has only gotten so far with DSRCT and Gabriel might not live to his 15th birthday! I can only imagine what Dr. Gomez will tell me tomorrow about Annabelle!"

"Michael. I only say this with the upmost respect—please remain calm. I know that you are upset and are channeling your anger on your children's doctors, but we are only here to help you and your children. We all here at the hospital will do anything possible to help combat these cancers. We will do any form of treatment we can find to help them. Please try to understand that. We are only here to help, Michael."

With tears in his eyes, Michael puts his head down. "Forgive me, Dr. Smith, but I just don't know what more I can do. I just have a bad feeling about what news I will hear tomorrow. I don't think I can take any more bad news. I just can't."

"I cannot say I understand where you are coming from, Michael, because I don't think anyone could understand unless they were in your shoes. I only know that in times like these, you should always look to our Father for answers."

"I do, doctor, but I am afraid that He isn't listening to me anymore."

"Michael, I have a friend here at the hospital who is a very good listener and is religious just like you. He is very discreet, and I think it would benefit you to give him a call—if not today, then after your visit with Dr. Gomez tomorrow. As you said yourself about news in threes, I am not supposed to say this as a doctor, but unfortunately, speaking from experience, I know that to be true. So, because you are feeling that tomorrow may not be good news, I ask that you please give him a call. Your children need you now more than ever. I see the fight in you. Just please never give up. If not for yourself, then call for your children's sake. Can you do that for me, Michael?"

"Yes, doctor, I can do that."

"I wish there were more that I could say, but that is all I have for you right now. Please take this card and go be with your children. Gabriel should be done by now."

"Thank you, doctor, for everything you are doing to help."

"It is my pleasure to help in any way possible. Again, Michael, I am very sorry that this is where we are now."

"Thank you, doctor."

"Remember to look to our Father for answers. Ask and He shall provide."

"That is the thing, doctor. I ask, but I still haven't received a response. I am going to be with Gabriel now. I promised him I would be there waiting for him."

"Take care, Michael. I've already sent his prescriptions to the pharmacy so you can pick them up on the way out."

"Thanks again, doctor. Take care." Michael leaves the doctor's office and makes his way to the treatment waiting room. Filled with emotions, he sits and says a prayer. "God, please give not only my children the strength to fight what's inside them, but please give me the strength to fight, as well."

The nurse then comes out. "Hi, Michael, Gabriel is finished with his treatment. He's been finished for some time now, but I knew you were with Dr. Smith, so I stayed with him to keep him company until you came back."

"Thank you, Pamela, and I apologize for my lateness."

"It's no problem at all, Michael. Besides, he is my little man. Did you get everything straightened out?"

"I did. I just needed to hear it a few times before I believed it to be true."

"Unfortunately, in these types of cases, some parents do."

"How is Gabriel feeling?"

"He is fatigued and feeling a little foggy-headed."

"That doesn't sound good."

"I understand your concern, Michael, but don't worry it is a normal side effect with this treatment. He will probably feel this way for some time today. It happens even to the most active children we see, and I know Gabriel is right up there on the active chart."

Michael smiles. "That he is, Pamela. Even though he has this illness, you would never guess it by the way he goes about his day."

"I will say this, Michael, he is a fighter—all of your children are."

"You are right on that, Pamela. Can he eat dinner or is it recommended that he not eat after his treatment?"

"No, he can have dinner. Dr. Smith already gave me his list to give to you. He wanted me to make sure that you know that Gabriel eats a variety of protein-rich foods that are low in fat like seafood, lean meat and poultry, Greek yogurt, eggs, beans, soy products, and unsalted nuts and seeds."

"Okay, I will make sure he eats those types of things. It shouldn't be a problem, because we already eat those types of meals with my girls' conditions."

"I was advised from their doctors to feed them protein-rich foods for their treatments as well. I just didn't know if Gabriel had to be on a specific diet."

"No, he just needs to watch foods that have fat in them, so no junk foods."

"Even though they are children, unfortunately they haven't had the opportunity to eat junk foods. They don't even know what fast food tastes like. I know I shouldn't say this as a father, but I wish that they got to experience what junk food tastes like."

"I know you do, Michael. I'm not speaking as a medical professional, but personally, I wish all children could have experiences like we did growing up like pigging out on foods that we knew weren't good for us and going to a fast food restaurant just to get the toys with the meals. But unfortunately some children are dealt with a hand that makes them no able to have experiences most children get to have. It breaks my heart to see that every day here."

"It breaks my heart as well, Pamela. And most children don't appreciate going to restaurants and snacking on junk foods while children in hospitals and those that have these illnesses around the world won't ever get a chance to experience what that is like. It's very sad to know that, but all these children that are with these illnesses, especially mine, don't see it that way because they feel sorry for normal children because they take advantage of life. I say that because of their actions, such as not going outside to play or not wanting to spend time with their families, and instead thinking they have something better to do with their time. Especially the fact that most children are buried into their phones these days and don't take the time to notice the world around them. I see it every day, but not my children or any children in hospitals that gets diagnosed with these illnesses—and I say illnesses not cancer because those children see it just as that: an illness. These amazing, brave children cherish every minute they can with their families and don't care about not being able to have things that other children have because they know how precious life is. I see it in my children, and I see it in this hospital."

"Wow, Michael, I knew you were a passionate person, but I had no idea you would say something like that."

They both smile.

I apologize for that. I kind of got off topic there for a minute. Now, about Gabriel...what else should I expect from his treatments?"

"No, that was very inspiring to hear you say. But yes, about Gabriel. He will most likely feel nauseous after his treatments, and don't be alarmed if he vomits. Although we know it is a side effect, feel free to contact us about any concern you may have."

"I always do."

"As you unfortunately know from your other children's treatments, there may be some symptoms afterwards such as constipation, taste changes, diarrhea, early satiety, dry or sore mouth, and as I told you, nausea. So make sure that he drinks plenty of fluids; he needs at least eight to ten eight-ounce glasses of liquids daily like water, fruit juices and nectars mixed with water, clear broth, sports drinks, and of course, there is always the drink that pediatricians recommend giving your children to stay hydrated, Kiddie Juice."

"Yeah, they can't get enough of that juice."

"I must tell you that Dr. Smith wants you to avoid things such as very hot or cold, high-sugar, high-fat, and even spicy foods. Those can be hard on his digestive system and may make his diarrhea worse if that is one of his symptoms, which it more than likely will be. The doctor also recommends that if Gabriel is having diarrhea, give him fruits and vegetables. Some things the doctor recommends giving him is well-cooked peeled and pureed or canned fruits and vegetables, bananas, peeled apples or applesauce, which works very well, juices or nectars mixed with water, of course, and even smooth peanut butter. Most of what he suggested to give him have potassium and liquid to help replace what his body loses from having diarrhea. The doctor also noted that those items have soluble fiber, which may decrease the symptom."

"As you just said, unfortunately, I know all about the symptoms from the girls' treatments. I have a list a mile long of different tips and tricks of foods and drinks to give them. When we first started all this medical stuff, Anna and I sat down with a nutritionist and along with their doctors' recommendations, and we went over what foods and drinks to give them. Of course, over the years, the list changes as they get older, but I pretty much have it down by now. But I really appreciate everything you all are doing here at the hospital for my children."

"It is our pleasure, Michael."

Michael looks at his watch. "Wow, I can't believe it's this late. I sometimes wonder where the time goes."

The nurse smiles. "As they say, time flies."

"My little buddy must be wondering where I am. I wonder why he hasn't asked for me yet."

"I can answer that. He is asleep. As I said, he is feeling fatigued, so I just let him sleep. That is why I came out here with you so we can discuss any questions you may have."

"I appreciate that, but is he alone?"

"No, no—he is in one of the after-treatment rooms we have for children that aren't able to leave immediately. He is in good hands."

"Okay, that's good, and thank you again for everything."

"You're welcome, Michael."

Michael then goes and gets Gabriel. "Hey buddy, time to wake up."

"Daddy… I beat up the meanies," Gabriel says groggily.

"I know you did, buddy. It's time to go home—only if you want to."

"Yeah… I'm sleepy."

"I know, buddy. Let's go home."

"Okay, Daddy."

Michael picks up Gabriel, and they meet up with Yolanda, Aunt Ruthie, Annabelle, and Jazmyn. "Hey ladies. Are we all set to go?"

"Yeah. What is wrong with bubby, Daddy? Why are you holding him?"

"He is very tired from the magic lasers, sweetie."

"Is my baby going to be okay?"

"Yes, Aunt Ruthie, he just needs rest. Yolanda, we need to pick up his medicines from the pharmacy on the way out."

"I will go get them, Michael."

"Do you remember where it's located?"

"I do. It's on the first floor, right?"

"Yes."

"Okay, while you all get in the car, I will pick up his prescriptions."

"Thank you, Yolanda."

"Michael, can I ask you something? Away from everyone…"

"Sure, sis. Aunt Ruthie, do you mind taking the girls to the car?"

"Of course, Michael."

"Thank you, Aunt Ruthie. Here are the keys."

"I will see you three soon. Let's go, babies."

"Okay, Aunt Ruthie."

"What do you need, Yolanda?"

"Is he sleeping?"

"Yes, he is exhausted."

"Aunt Ruthie and I noticed that something is different in your eyes when you first walked up to us."

"Let's walk and talk."

They begin to walk down to the pharmacy.

"What happened in there?"

"I don't know how to say this, but I was wrong about everything."

"What do you mean?"

"We weren't getting tests results today, and Gabriel wasn't getting his treatment on suspicion alone. He has DSRCT, Yolanda."

Yolanda gasps. "Oh, my Lord, no!"

"I'm afraid so. And, apparently, I knew all along. I just reacted the same way I did when Annabelle and Jazmyn were diagnosed. I didn't want to believe it was true."

"What does this mean, Michael?"

"It means, Yolanda, that now my little buddy here," Michael says with tears in his eyes, "has a very small chance to live to see his 15th birthday, and he will be very lucky if he lives that long."

"What are they going to do for him?"

"That's the thing, Yolanda, there is nothing they can do at this point. Because it is so rare, they have very little information on it."

"Michael, what are you going to do?"

"The only thing that I can do, Yolanda, at this point, is to pray. After hearing the news about Jazmyn yesterday and Gabriel today..." Michael fights his tears. "Yolanda, I already received a text from Dr. Gomez that she needs to speak to me tomorrow, and I am deeply afraid to hear what news she has for me about..." Michael's tears begin to fall down his cheek, "... Annabelle."

Chapter 8

"Michael…Michael…"

Michael rolls over. "Yes, sis, what is it?"

"It's time to get up."

"What time is it?"

"It's 8 in the morning."

Michael jumps up out of bed. "What?! I am always up at 6:30 in the morning! I know because I set the alarm, or did I?"

"You did, but after how quiet you were yesterday when we came home and how quiet you were during dinner, Aunt Ruthie and I decided to let you sleep in today. We both know for a fact that you didn't sleep that well last night."

"I appreciate the gesture, Yolanda, but I do not have time to sleep in. I am on a tight schedule as it is. I need to get breakfast for the children, make sure they read, get their medicines ready… I just do not have time to waste."

"Michael, it is all taken care of. I made breakfast, and before you ask, yes, I did go by the list of foods and drinks they can have. While I was cooking,

Aunt Ruthie made sure the cuties read something and I know you like to double-check their medicines, but I already did. You know you always sort out their medicines on Sundays for the week. Don't worry—it's all taken care of. Now get dressed because your cuties are asking for you and they want to eat, and you know they don't like to eat without you. So get up because breakfast is ready."

"Okay, thank you, Yolanda. Go ahead and serve them and tell them that I am coming out. Give me about 10 minutes or less and I will be out there with you all."

"Sure thing, Michael."

"Oh, one more thing. Please remember that they say grace before they eat."

"I will, Michael."

"Okay. Thank you, Yolanda." Michael then gets showered, dressed, and heads out to dining room table where everyone is waiting on him.

"Daddy!" the children shout as they run up to him.

"Good morning, soldiers, and how are we today?"

"My tummy hurts a little today."

"I know, sweetie, but you go in for your magic potion to beat up the mean-ies. Thank you for telling me. Gabriel, I know you were very tired and felt sick last night. How are you feeling, buddy?"

"I feel better, but I can't stop pooping."

Michael smiles. "I know, buddy, but that is why Aunt Yolanda made a special breakfast for you. To help with that. Your doctor gave you some medicines to help with some things that you will feel after you get magic lasers."

"Okay, Daddy."

"How is my princess today?"

"Princess!"

"That's my girl. Good morning, Aunt Ruthie. How are you doing this morning?"

"I am doing good, but I need to ask how you are feeling, Michael."

"I am better, Aunt Ruthie, but I suggest asking me again tonight after our trip to Adventure Land."

"I will, Michael. Believe me, I will."

"Anyways, breakfast looks good, Yolanda. I can't thank you both enough for what you two did this morning. Although I am a little upset, I know your hearts were in the right places."

"Hush now, Michael. It was our pleasure to spend some quality time with these babies."

"I know you must be not to thrilled about what we did, but you must look at it from our perspective, Michael. You needed to get some rest."

"I understand that, Yolanda, but I don't like to waste any minute I have with these soldiers. But I must say that you two did a very good job. I will be honest with you ladies and say that it kind of makes me feel dispensable."

"Don't be silly, Michael, we could never replace you. Now, get you a plate and come sit with us because the children have a question about faith, and Aunt Ruthie and I cannot wait to hear what you say to them."

"I will say this, Yolanda, if, God forbid, anything happens to me, I can at least take comfort that you and Aunt Ruthie will be able to take care of these soldiers. I only say that in talking so I don't want to hear anything on the subject. I will say that there is no one I trust with my soldiers more than you two ladies." Michael smiles and gets himself a plate for food and sits down at the table.

"Okay, so what is this question about faith?"

"Well, Daddy, bubby and I overheard Aunt Ruthie and Yolanda saying that your faith was being tested and how you need to find your faith again more than anything right now. So…"

"Okay, continue. I'm listening."

"Bubby, you ask Daddy."

"Just come out with it, soldiers."

"Daddy, what does that mean that you need to find your faith again? Where did you lose it?"

"Well, buddy, first allow me to say this—I did not expect that to be something you all would be worried about, but Daddy is kind of lost now. You all here know I will always be honest with you, so here it is."

Everyone leans in to hear Michael speak.

"I always have faith in the Lord, knowing he has a plan for us all here on Earth, but as of late, my faith is being tested by things that are happening to you soldiers that I can't get into now. God does not play games with us, and tests of faiths are just to see if we believe in Him. He has his reasons for doing everything that He does for us. So, as a believer, you may not understand why certain things are happening in your lives, but you must trust God in everything that He does for you. He loves us so much that he will not allow you to go through situations in your lives if you are not able to handle it.

"There is going to be a point in your lives when you start to question the things that are happening in this world and in your lives. Some always say if they were to ask God one question it would be why bad things happen to good people. I, myself, cannot answer that question, nor can anyone here on Earth. It is all about faith and trusting in God that he will always be there for you."

"Like Jesus is, Daddy?"

"Exactly, buddy. All of heaven is watching over us, making sure we are okay here on Earth. God knows why certain things happen to people who feel that they don't deserve what happens to them, but most people don't see all the wonderful things that God has blessed us with. Some are going through certain situations in their lives and only singling them out instead of thanking God for the good things that are happening."

"Like what, Daddy?"

"Well, sweetie, there are such things like waking up in the morning, seeing your family's beautiful faces every day, feeling the warmth of a hug from someone you care about, having clothes to wear, somewhere to bathe, shower, and rest. You see, many don't notice those because some don't look at them as blessings. They think they're just another thing that they have. Every minute we have on this Earth to experience things like feeling the love for one other is a blessing. Unfortunately, bad things do happen in this world to very loving people, but it's not for us to understand why. We must always have faith in our Lord. I feel that faith isn't just about how much you believe in the Lord, but how much faith you have in your fellow brother and sister."

"I have faith in bubby, Daddy."

"I have faith in sissy too, Daddy."

Michael smiles. "That is very sweet of both of you to say, but what I meant by that is your fellow brother and sister in the world. I will explain. You see, as I told you all yesterday, we all were created with the same blood, so that means that we are all brothers and sisters in this world. God gave us the power of love so that we may love one another and help each other out. No one can force you to have faith or give it to you; it's something that you yourself must have. I thank God that I was tasked with instilling faith to you all, but I cannot make you have faith. That is something between you and God. I can only try to teach you all the best way possible."

"Can you tell us in like a story like you always do, Daddy?"

"I will, buddy. Okay, pretend life is an ocean. We all are captains of our own ships, just floating on this ocean. We get the privilege of deciding where we want to go because God gave us free will. Is everyone with me so far?"

"Yes," everyone says, listening in.

"So, by God allowing us to go where we want, it's then up to us to pick our destinations. Some unfortunate people jump off the ship because the ocean is too much for them to handle. Some only search for treasure, and although they do end up finding it on their journey, they don't realize they are all alone on a deserted island, because they left everyone behind in order to get it. Then you have the rest of us who drift along the ocean in search of one day finding the promised land. In case I am losing you all, it represents heaven. So, we go through our journeys, drifting along the ocean in hopes of one day finding it.

"Now, the thing about that is that we do see land in the distance, but most people try to take the easy route and don't see the dangers of the waters. Most rush, thinking that they have everything it takes to land safely on the promised land. Most, however, are wrong because they don't notice the dangers in the ocean like rocks, and they crash their ships and come up short. You see, what I am trying to tell you all is... first let me ask you guys this so I know you all are with me. What guides boats safely to shore?"

"A flag?"

"No, buddy."

"A pole?"

"No, sweetie."

"I know, Michael—a lighthouse."

"You are right, Aunt Ruthie. So, on to the story. Many—and I say many—of us are tired of drifting on the ocean and just think all they have to do to get to the promised land is just steer their ships, but that is not the case. You see, soldiers, many fail to see that in order to safely land, you must follow the light. And who is the light?"

"God?" the children ask.

"Good job, soldiers. Now, just as a lighthouse never leaves its position, neither does God. He is always there, shining ever so brightly, guiding us to safety. All we must do is follow him. Many think they are too far away to reach the light, and they think that the light keeps moving farther and farther away from them. I am here to tell you all that, as humans, we fail to see that it is us who drifts away from the light because he never leaves us. He is always there waiting for us to see his light shining so that we may safely land. To make it more amazing, soldiers, God had put a safety device, a life preserver, in our boats because years and years ago, God saw that we weren't all safely coming to land. So he put that life preserver in our boats to save us in our time of need. Who am I talking about?"

"Just tell us, Daddy! We want to know who it is!"

"Okay, sweetie. It was Jesus."

"Wow! Jesus, Daddy?"

"That's right, buddy, because God loves this world so much that he gave Jesus to us so that we may come home. Now, when you do see the lighthouse that will guide you to the promised land, you can't just bring the ship onto shore right?"

"No!" say the children loudly.

"Exactly, soldiers. Although there will be storms on your journey, and you will sometimes feel that the light isn't there anymore, you must always remain faithful that the light is there, shining ever so brightly, waiting for you to come home. So, when the time comes for you to one day get off your ship, all you need is your faith that you will get there, the lighthouse, and the life preserver that has been with you the whole time, and together, you may safely arrive onto the promised land. So always obey and follow God, have faith that He is always there, and accept Jesus Christ as your Lord and Savior.

"You know from your Bible readings that Jesus clearly stated in John 14:6, 'I am the way and the truth and the life. No one comes to the Father except through me.' That is very powerful, soldiers, because we have a chance to be with our Father and Lord and Savior in the kingdom of heaven, but you must remember to also have faith. Until now, I thought it was God who was drifting from me, but thanks to you all caring so much about me to ask about faith I realize that it is I who am drifting from God because of the meanies in you soldiers. I want to apologize to you all for doing so."

"Daddy, I love it when you tell us stories."

"Me too, Daddy."

"Thank you, soldiers, and I am always happy to tell them to you all. Looks like you soldiers are done eating. Time for you-know-what."

"Yeah, yeah, we know."

"Sissy, you can go first since today you go in for magic potion, and like Daddy says, ladies first."

"Thank you, bubby."

Michael, filled with pride, smiles. "I am so proud to be your father, soldiers. Okay, sweetie, here is your cup."

"Thank you."

"You are welcome. And here is yours, buddy."

"Thank you, Daddy."

"You are very welcome, buddy. Princess, I didn't forget about you. Here is yours."

"'Kay."

"I know that is your way of saying thank you, so you are welcome, princess."

"All gone, Daddy."

"Mine is empty too, Daddy."

"Okay, soldiers, you know what's next."

"Okay," Annabelle and Gabriel say, leaving to go get dressed to leave.

"So, ladies what did you think of today's speech?"

"It was very moving, Michael."

"I agree with Yolanda. I just love hearing you break down your definitions into metaphors for your babies."

Michael smiles. "Well, thank you, ladies. To be honest, I thought it was a little preachy. I didn't know if I had gotten the message out clearly enough.

I should have just told them the concept of the story instead of talking from my soapbox again."

"Don't ever say that, Michael. I can't speak for Yolanda, but I just love it when you talk in metaphors."

"I agree with Aunt Ruthie. It's very interesting the way you speak."

Michael smiles. "Don't think I don't know what happened today."

"What are you talking about, Michael?"

"Yes, Michael whatever do you mean?"

Yolanda and Aunt Ruthie smile deviously at each other.

"Uh huh, ladies. Just know that I am on to you two, but out of all sincerity, I want to thank both of you for keeping me in check. Even though I may seem out of it with everything that has happened and what is going to happen today, it's always a good feeling when you and my soldiers pull me back in. Unfortunately, I just have a strong feeling that today isn't going to be a good day either, but I can take comfort in knowing my family is always here to save me. I always think to myself that I have seen and been through it all and that I can handle anything that comes my way, but I never imagined that I would be losing my faith."

"That's why we are here, Michael—for you and those cuties."

"Exactly, Michael, and as you said, God puts certain people in our lives to help guide us through our troubles."

"I know that, Yolanda, Aunt Ruthie, and I am grateful that I have you all in my lives. It's just I don't think I can handle any more news. That reminds me—Dr. Smith gave me a number to one of his friends who works at the hospital and claims that he is a very good listener, but I know he is a therapist who works with parents of children with cancers."

"So, what are you waiting for?"

"I agree with Yolanda. I don't see why you haven't called yet. I am sorry to say this, Michael, but you are way overdue to talk to someone. Especially to a professional."

"Don't get me wrong, I appreciate what you two and everyone at the hospital are trying to do by getting me to sit down and talk to someone, but I don't think anyone can help me at this point. I always pride myself on being tough and strong for my soldiers, but I must admit I have weakened at this point in my life, and I am afraid that I am too far gone to help."

"That right there is reason enough, Michael, for you sit down with someone and talk your problems through."

"I will be more direct than Yolanda. Michael, you may believe that you are this big, strong, macho person who can handle anything because you claim to have seen and been through it all, but you seem to forget that you are human. You have so much on your plate that it breaks my heart to see you losing your faith. I don't know why you didn't speak to a professional when Annabelle was first diagnosed, because no human on earth can handle hearing that their child has cancer, and you have three, Michael. Three! Not only with cancers but rare cancers and that is way too much for someone to take on by themselves."

"Aunt Ruthie, forgive me for saying this, but what can anyone do for me at this point? What good will it do? It certainly won't take their illnesses away. I just don't see the point. Besides, I have you two ladies to talk to."

"Don't make jokes, Michael, because I am serious right now. You need to sit down with someone. If not the therapist, then at least speak with a minister. I am afraid for your soul because of the way you keep saying that God isn't listening to you. You know that God is always with you. I love you like a son, Michael, and I would love to think when this world is done and over with, we all will be in heaven together. I see you going down a dark path, and I fear for your soul."

"I appreciate and hear everything you both are saying, but my soul is something you never have to worry about. Although these days are darker than most, I will always remain faithful in the Lord and his plans. I just wanted to tell you both that it was just talk, I meant what I said about trusting you both with my soldiers if I were no longer here."

"I don't want to hear you speak like that, Michael."

"I am with Aunt Ruthie on that."

"No, please, I want both of you to listen to me, because we never get a chance to speak about it. With what happened with Anna and the way we weren't prepared, I want to get this out there. If, God forbid, something does happen to me at any point, I ask that you both take care of them."

"Michael—"

He interrupts. "No, please, Yolanda, let me finish. There is no one else who knows my children like you both do. They respect and love you both, and I know that if I were ever to leave this beautiful world to enter another, they would be in good hands. I should have told you this way back, but we never had an opportunity to discuss it. I have an insurance policy that will take care of everything. This house is paid for, and although I will leave it to the soldiers, Aunt Ruthie, Yolanda, it will transfer in your names."

"I don't want to hear anymore, Michael."

"Aunt Ruthie, please allow me to finish."

"Michael, I don't like this kind of conversation, and besides, don't you need us to sign something?"

Michael smiles. "Do you both remember signing those documents a while ago?"

"I do. I remember it was like signing a contract or something."

"As do I. There were so many forms to fill out."

"Well, I'm sorry, ladies, to tell you that that was sort of my insurance policy just in case something were to happen to me. Did you two ever wonder why you both have access to the soldiers' medical records and are able to get their medicines? Why I showed you which medicines and at which time they can take them? Why I even have a schedule and their lists of foods and drinks right there on the fridge? Why their doctors know who you two are? Did neither one of you ever wonder why I ask both of you to do little things around here, and no, I don't mean cleaning; I mean by making sure they read, say grace, get their baths, and say their prayers at night?"

"We love doing those things for those babies of yours."

"I'm with Aunt Ruthie on that, and besides, sometimes you're busy, Michael."

"Yes, Yolanda, I am, but I am never too busy for those tasks. I am just ensuring that no matter what God has planned for me, my children are in very capable hands. Before you say anything, Aunt Ruthie, I know you can never in a million years guess what God has planned for us. I am just doing what any parent would do for their children to make sure that if something were to happen they would be well taken care of. I carry on about definitions of different topics in front of you both because you two can carry on what I teach to my children. I know you two do not like what I am saying now but you both must understand that if—and I only say if—something were to happen to me, I could smile from above knowing that my children would be fine down here on Earth with you two. Now I know both of you have comments you would like to make, but remember, this is just me talking. I must get princess here dressed and make sure we all are ready to leave soon. Once again, I know I ran my mouth as usual, but please respect what I am saying to you both."

"Daddy... princess."

"I know, princess. Let's get you dressed."

"'Kay."

"Michael, don't think you will just say your piece and we'll be done. We will talk about this again."

"You heard Aunt Ruthie, Michael. Now go make sure those cuties are ready to leave soon."

"Okay ladies." Michael then gets Jazmyn dressed and waits by the door. "Okay soldiers, you both had plenty of time getting ready. What is taking so long?

Gabriel comes to the door. "I'm ready, Daddy, but sissy said her tummy hurts."

"Yolanda!"

"I'm right here, Michael. What do you need?"

"Annabelle is in pain. Can you take princess here and get everyone in the car for me? And one more thing, if you don't mind, please start the car for me."

"Of course, Michael. Aunt Ruthie, it's time to leave!"

"Okay, I'm coming!"

"Oh, Yolanda can you double-check their bags for me?"

"Already have, Michael. As I told you we covered everything this morning."

"Thank you."

"Okay, cuties, let's go get in the car."

"Okay," Gabriel says, walking out as Michael goes to Annabelle.

Hey, sweetie, are you okay?"

"Yeah I am, but my tummy hurts, Daddy."

"I know it does, Annabelle, but you know you are going in for your magic potion to feel better."

"I know. It's just that I hate when the meanies make me feel this way."

"I know, sweetie, and so do I, but we must leave because it's almost time. I will wait with you if you need me to, sweetie. We will only leave when you are able to."

"No, it's okay. I really need to get my magic potion to beat up these meanies."

"Are you sure, sweetie?"

"Yeah, I am definitely sure that I am ready."

"Okay, sweetie, let's go if you are ready. Aunt Yolanda has your bag in the car."

"Okay, Daddy."

"Let me just set the alarm and lock this door." He does so. "Okay, sweetie. Looks like we are set to go to Adventure Land for your magic potion."

Michael and Annabelle get in the car. "Everyone buckled in?

"Yes!" Everyone shouts. They then get on the road.

"Okay, time for Adventure Land."

"Yay!" Gabriel says loudly. "Sissy, are you not happy we are going to Adventure Land?"

"I am, bubby. My tummy just hurts."

"It's okay, sissy. Like you told me yesterday, you are going to feel all better after you get your magic potion, and you are going to kick those meanies' butts!"

"I know, bubby. Thank you."

"You're welcome, sissy."

Michael, listening to what he hears, is filled with pride. "You know, buddy, what your sister needs from you?"

"What?"

"One of your special hugs."

"Oh, sissy, I am going to give you a big special hug before you go in for your magic potion."

"That will be nice, bubby."

They then arrive at the hospital.

"Look sissy! Adventure Land!"

"Okay."

"Buddy, she is just hurting from the meanies. Okay everyone, let's go in yet again."

They enter the hospital and take the elevator to the children's floor and arrive.

"Okay, Yolanda, Aunt Ruthie, you both know the drill by now, so must I repeat it?"

"No, we know what to do with these babies."

"Yolanda, are you all set?"

"Yes, Michael, just make sure your cutie gets the treatment she needs, and whatever the doctor tells you, do not lose your cool."

"I can't make any promises, but I hear you, sis. Please remember to give Gabriel his medicine to help him with his stomach."

"Way ahead of you, Michael."

"Okay, buddy, you know what your sister needs from you before you all leave us."

"Oh yeah." Gabriel runs up to Annabelle and gives her a big hug. "There you are, sissy. That will help you fight the meanies."

"Thank you, bubby. Daddy, my chest feels weird again."

"It does?!"

"Yes."

"Okay, sweetie. Have a seat and rest for a few minutes and tell me what the problem is." He goes and sits her down.

"It just feels like someone is standing on my chest."

"Yolanda, please go tell Stephanie that Dr. Gomez needs to come out immediately."

"Right away, Michael."

Yolanda rushes to the check-in desk.

"Daddy, it hurts."

Michael, with concern, yells to the receptionist, "Stephanie, get any doctor out here please!"

Stephanie comes to them. "What's going on with Annabelle, Michael?"

"She says her chest hurts."

"I've already paged the doctor that she needs assistance."

A nurse comes out. "The doctor is coming out, Michael. Annabelle, I need you to tell me what is going on with you."

"My chest feels weird."

Dr. Gomez comes. "What seems to be the problem?"

"She says her chest feels weird, doctor."

"I think it's her angina, but she hasn't done any activities to cause this!"

"Michael, please remain calm. Annabelle, how does your chest feel weird?"

"It feels like someone is stepping on it. It hurts."

"Doctor, what is going on?"

The doctor begins examining her.

"Does your arm hurt?"

"No."

"How long have you felt like this?"

"Just now."

"It has been at least a couple minutes since she first told me, doctor."

"Is it going away, Annabelle?"

"Yeah, it doesn't feel weird like it did."

"Nurse, call for transport to take her down to run tests. I will send the orders down."

"Yes, doctor."

"What is going on, doctor?"

"She doesn't appear to have had a heart attack or anything of that nature, but I want to run tests to ensure that everything is working like it should be."

"Why is this happening to someone so young?"

"Michael, I believe it is her angina, but I want to get these tests done to make sure."

"I want to make sure she is going to be okay, doctor. I don't like these guessing games."

"Neither do I, Michael. Don't worry, from what I can see it's the angina that is causing this."

The transport comes to pick up Annabelle, and the nurse helps her up.

"Okay, Annabelle, ready to go for a ride?"

"Yeah. Daddy, are you coming with me?"

"Dr. Gomez can I go with her?"

"No, she will be mainly getting tests done. Don't worry, she is in good hands."

"Daddy must wait here for you, but I will be right here when you get back, okay?"

"Okay, Daddy."

"Don't worry, you have some special people that will be right there with you."

"Okay."

They take Annabelle away.

"Dr. Gomez, please tell me what is happening with my daughter."

"Michael, I need for her to get the tests done before I can discuss it further."

"You sent me a text yesterday saying that you needed to see me today. So why can't we discuss that matter?"

"I still need to speak with you, but the episode she just had changes our conversation entirely. I know you don't want to hear this, but don't worry. Once I get the tests results back, I will sit down with you, and at that time, I will explain everything to you."

"What about her treatment?"

"I need to clear her first before she can undergo treatment."

"I care most of all for her wellbeing, but she really needs her treatment, doctor. She is so much pain from the cancer."

"I understand that, Michael, and when I can clear her to receive treatment, I will, but only if I feel she will be able to withstand it."

"I understand, doctor. Thank you."

"Don't worry. Annabelle will be back before you know it. I will see you soon, Michael."

"Thank you, doctor."

The doctor leaves, and Michael goes to his family that is waiting.

"Daddy?"

"Yes buddy?"

"Is sissy going to be okay?"

"Of course she is, buddy, don't you worry about a thing."

"Where did she go?"

"Well, buddy, she went to get some tests done."

"But sissy isn't in school."

Michael smiles. "No, buddy. She went to get pictures done, and most likely they are going to get a little blood from her."

"Oh okay."

"I tell you what. How about Aunt Ruthie and Aunt Yolanda take you and princess to the playroom or the sports room that you like so much."

"Can we, Aunt Ruthie?"

"Of course we can, Gabriel! Anything for my little babies."

"Yay!" Gabriel says, excited.

"Yolanda, are you coming?"

"No, Aunt Ruthie, if you don't mind, I am going to stay and talk with Michael, if that is okay."

"It's okay, Yolanda, I can wait here by myself."

"Hush Michael."

"I don't mind at all. Besides, I will be happy to have these babies all to myself. Let's go, babies."

"Okay," Gabriel says, waving goodbye as they leave.

"I will see you soon guys!"

"Michael, while we have time, let's talk."

"You know I love you, Yolanda, but I don't think I will be very talkative with what just happened."

"Well, let's start with that first. What is going through your mind?"

"You don't want to know."

"Yes, Michael, I asked because I don't want to know," she says sarcastically. "You can tell me. It's just you and me here."

"For one, I am just thinking about Annabelle and what could have caused her to feel that way. She didn't run, walk fast, or anything that would make her chest do that, and I am just trying to figure out why."

"Like Dr. Gomez said, she wants Annabelle to get the tests done before she can sit down with you."

"That's what I am afraid of, Yolanda. I can only imagine what she will tell me. I know it's not going to be good news."

"I didn't know you could tell the future. Quick, tell me the lotto numbers!" she said jokingly as Michael smiles.

"Quit it, Yolanda."

"Okay, I will. But on a serious note, Michael, you are not a psychic, so why must you think things will be terrible?"

"You heard what the doctor said. She did want to speak to me but after what happened to Annabelle that conversation has changed. In my experience, it's not good when a doctor says that."

"That may be the case, Michael, but quit putting yourself through so much turmoil over things that haven't happened yet."

"Yolanda, I didn't go to school to be a doctor, but from what I know with my children, it's never a good sign when a doctor calls you into his or her office."

"I know you have been through so much with your children, and I know it's more than most people go through in their lifetime, but you are right— you are not a doctor. So why must you think negatively? Sure, it's easy for anyone to tell you to quit driving yourself crazy about what might happen, especially those who are not in your shoes. But don't worry, I am not going to tell you to that, but I will say this: you must stay with your faith and trust in our Father to help you and your children."

"I will be honest with you. I am a faithful, God-loving man, and I always look to our Father for guidance. It's just that I pray and pray over again to save and heal my children and to give me the strength to guide them to safety, but…" Michael puts his head down. "I am afraid he isn't listening to my prayers."

"How can you say that, Michael? You know for a fact that God hears our prayers. Just look around you."

"Yolanda, I hate myself for saying this, but indeed, look around you. Where are we?"

"We are in Adventure Land."

"No, Yolanda, we are in a hospital."

"Michael, you created Adventure Land for your children, and I have never heard you say this place was a hospital," Yolanda says with a concerned look.

"Forgive me, Yolanda, but we are indeed in a hospital because there is sickness everywhere here. Children are dying every day from their illnesses. To make it worse, some that don't make it are either my children's ages or younger, and my soldiers knew some of them by name! I just don't understand why there is so much pain in this world. Why many children must suffer. It's just not fair."

"Michael, no one can begin to understand what you are feeling, but please don't give up. You are the most wonderful, caring person I know. Especially the way you created Adventure Land for your children. You turned this hospital into a theme park when most parents would have been more terrified than their children, but not you. Unfortunately, yes, your children must come here more times than you would like them to, but it was you who had created this wonderful imaginative world for your children to be safe in, and it is breaking my heart to hear you speak this way."

"For the record, it wasn't just me that had created this world for my soldiers. It was—or I should say is—a collective effort from all the great people here at the hospital and the wonderful things they do here that helped create Adventure Land. Especially the way they helped me call their treatments 'magic potions' and 'magic lasers'. I know I am out of line for saying everything I said, but I just don't know what more I can do. I am hanging on by a thread. I keep praying to our Father for guidance, but I honestly feel like I am alone here."

"You are never alone, Michael. Not only Aunt Ruthie and I are here with you, but so is our Father. You tell us all the time how blessed you are for having such a wonderful family. How blessed you are with the staff and people here at this hospital—or should I say Adventure Land—that are here for your children and many more that are going through these illnesses. God is always with you, Michael. Our Father is with us all, and you know this because you tell us that every day. Or is that something that you have forgotten?"

"No, I didn't forget that. Yolanda, I know our Father is with us, and yes, I truly believe God is with us every day. Just by the blessings we receive every day alone are indication that our Father is always there with us."

"By you knowing that then why do you feel alone?"

"My children are suffering Yolanda. I don't know how many times I must tell you that I pray constantly on their wellbeing and the world's, at that. It's just that I see so much going on with my children and in this world, and my only thought as a human being is why? Before you say anything, yes, I have faith and believe in our Father, but I am only human. I know God has a plan for us all, and I say this to you guys all the time—it's not for our understanding of why things happen in this world, but I just would like God to hear my prayers to save and heal my children. I would love for an opportunity to talk to our Father and for him to tell me what his will is."

"Any person would love to jump on that opportunity, but you must understand that our Father is always with us and He will never leave us alone. You must remain faithful. As you told us in the story today, God loves us so much that he gave us a life preserver in our boats to safely get home. I think it's time for you to use it because, as in your metaphor, you are drowning now in the sea of life."

Michael smiles. "Why must you use my own metaphor against me?"

Yolanda smiles. "Because I love you so much that I know the way you are feeling about God. This isn't like you."

"Thank you for everything you just said to me. I do have faith in our Father, but to be honest, I still don't know what more I can do."

"Pray, Michael. Just pray. That is all you can do."

"Thank you, Yolanda, and for the record I am truly blessed to have you as my sister."

They both smile at each other.

"Well, thank you, Michael. That means a lot coming from you."

"I wonder where Annabelle could be. It seems like an eternity waiting here like this."

"Be patient, Michael. You know she is in good hands here."

"I know that, Yolanda. I still don't understand why I couldn't go down with her."

"She is getting tests done, Michael, and knowing you, you would have just been in the way."

They both laugh.

"Yeah, I must admit, you do have a point. I wonder how Aunt Ruthie is doing with my little buddy and princess."

"Knowing her, she is having a good time with them. She loves those cuties. So do I. You know this by the way she calls them her babies."

"You are right about that. I tell you this, I know Aunt Ruthie is getting a workout keeping up with my little soldiers."

They both laugh.

"Yeah, more than likely she is."

As more time passes by, Michael grows impatient. "Where is Annabelle?"

"Michael, the doctor said she would be back before you know it."

"Yolanda, I am a patient person, and you know I do not rush things, especially when it comes to medical procedures, but it is going on over four hours now since Annabelle went down to get tests done."

"It takes time, and you know how great this place is. I am sure they are just covering all bases before allowing her to get her treatment."

"You're right. I apologize."

"Quit apologizing for everything, Michael. You are a concerned father. You are allowed to be concerned over your children." Yolanda notices the nurse. "Look, Michael, there is the nurse coming now."

Michael and Yolanda both get up.

"Hi Michael."

"Where is Annabelle?"

"She is sleeping. She was in pain, so the doctor gave her some pain medicines."

"Without my consent?"

"Michael, I understand as a parent how that may upset you, but you gave Dr. Gomez and the hospital permission to treat Annabelle any way possible. It was in the consent form that you signed."

"I apologize, nurse. It's just that my nerves are bad now, and I am just worried about Annabelle."

"You don't ever have to apologize, Michael. I completely understand."

"Did Dr. Gomez clear Annabelle for treatment?"

"Unfortunately, no she didn't."

"What is the problem?"

"You must speak with Dr. Gomez about that. She is waiting for you in her office."

"Oh Lord, here we go again."

Yolanda speaks up. "Michael, remember what we talked about. Whatever it is, just remain calm."

"Okay, sis. Nurse, what about Annabelle's treatment? She is in pain."

"That is why the doctor gave her pain medicines to help her cope with the pain. Don't worry. She is resting comfortably."

"I appreciate that, but I don't want to leave her in there by herself."

"I will stay with my cutie, Michael. You go and sit down with Dr. Gomez. And whatever the discussion is, remember what we talked about: have faith."

"Okay Yolanda. Thank you."

"Nurse, can you take me to Annabelle?"

"Sure, right this way."

As Yolanda and the nurse leave, Yolanda turns to Michael.

"Remember, Michael…"

"I will, Yolanda."

They both leave, and Michael goes to the doctor's office.

"Lord, give me strength." He knocks. "Doctor Gomez?"

The door opens. "Hi Michael, please come in and sit."

"Forgive me, doctor, but I am starting to hate those words."

"I know you are, Michael."

Michael sits down nervously.

"How are things at home?"

"Just fine. Well, for the most part. We have our routines down—medicines, watch what they eat, say our prayers, you know, the usual."

"That's good, Michael."

"Look, Dr. Gomez, I really do appreciate you asking me how things are going, but I know you didn't bring me in here to talk about how things are going at home."

"You are right, Michael, I didn't. But I always want to make sure that you yourself are okay."

"I apologize, doctor. I was out of line."

"No, Michael, you weren't. Of course you are concerned about Annabelle, and I have yet to see a parent who walks into my office calmly. Although you are very different than most parents I come across, by the way. You created Adventure Land for your children. You are still a parent, Michael."

"I realize that, doctor, but it was you all here that helped. Now, on to Annabelle. Please don't beat around the bush. Just please tell me what is going on with my little girl."

"Of course, Michael. I ran tests focusing mainly on her heart, and I am afraid to say the results don't look good."

"Meaning what, doctor?"

"Annabelle is having heart complications."

"What?!"

"Any patient with heart complications is cause for concern, but in Annabelle's case, because she has progeria, it doesn't look good for her."

"She is so young; how can she have heart complications?"

"She is strong Michael, but she does have a rare cancer, and now with her heart problems, it does not appear to be good for Annabelle."

"She is only 12 years old, doctor! How can this be happening?"

"It's because of her age, Michael. You yourself know what the life expectancy is in a child with progeria."

"Her birthday is in three days, doctor! I just assumed it's a miracle that she gets to celebrate her 13th birthday."

"It is a miracle that she made it this far, Michael. Especially the way she is now. Normally I see patients with progeria in worse conditions than she is now. Someone up there is looking out for her, but you know what the life expectancy is, and unfortunately, it's only thirteen years."

"Wait a minute, doctor. I know I may not be the smartest man, but what are you trying to say?"

"Michael, I need you to prepare."

"Prepare for what, doctor?!"

"With the shape her heart is in, Michael, I am very sorry to tell you this, but it will be a miracle if Annabelle makes it to her birthday."

"What?! That can't be true, doctor! Just look at Annabelle! Yes, she may have a high-pitched voice, and she may not look like children her age, but she is one of the most wonderful, loving, happy children out there! She does not look like someone who is on the verge of succumbing to her illness."

"Her spirit may not say so, but unfortunately, Michael, her body does."

"What do we do from here?"

"I personally would like Annabelle to remain here, Michael, but because she is a strong, spirited child and there is no need for her being here, it's your call."

"Which is best for her health?"

"Unfortunately, neither one will be. It's just nature taking its course. No matter where Annabelle is, Michael, if God says it's her time, that is when it will be."

"Oh Lord, no!"

"Michael, I am very sorry for what is happening. I will give you medicines to help her feel comfortable at home if that is what you want to do."

"Just tell me this. Will it be dangerous to take her home?"

"No, Michael. I don't understand it, but just by the way Annabelle's spirit is, you will never know that she is going through these problems or even that she has progeria. It's a miracle."

"No, doctor, all my children are miracles, but unfortunately now..." Michael's tears begin to fall. "I am staring down death again."

"I am very sorry, Michael."

"What can I do, doctor?"

"All you can do is cherish every moment, not only with Annabelle, but with your other children as well."

"When can I take Annabelle home?"

"Since she had the episode, she became a patient, but I will discharge her immediately."

"Thank you, doctor." "You're welcome, Michael, and again, I am very sorry."

"I can't let my family see me like this."

"It's understandable, Michael. You can take all the time you need in my office to compose yourself."

"Thank you, doctor. Thank you for everything."

"You never need to say thank you. It's why we are here. I wish things could turn out better for all my patients, but unfortunately, God has other plans."

"That is what scares me, doctor."

"Take all the time you need, Michael, and please don't hesitate to call me or the hospital for any reason."

Michael wipes is tears. "Thank you, doctor."

"Goodbye, Michael."

The doctor leaves and Michael shouts to heaven. "Lord, where are you?! Why is this happening to such loving children?!" Michael drops his head and softly says, "Why is this happening to me?" He sits there for a while in silence, then composes himself and goes to Annabelle's room.

"Daddy…" Annabelle says groggily.

"Its's okay, sweetie. I know you are tired."

"I want to go home."

"Okay, sweetie, we may leave when you are ready to."

Yolanda sees that something is wrong with Michael. "Michael, what did you and Dr. Gomez discuss?"

Michael knew in his heart that he could not tell anyone what he and the doctor had discussed. "I will never lie to you, Yolanda, but trust me when I say this, it's nothing for you to be concerned about."

"What does that mean?"

"I am saying that we must have faith, Yolanda. Remember?"

"Okay, Michael. If you say so."

"Sweetie, the doctor said you may leave when you are ready to."

"I just want to go home, Daddy."

"Okay sweetie. We can."

"Okay."

"Yolanda, can you do me a favor and go get her medicines from the pharmacy and round up the troops?"

"Sure Michael."

"We will meet you all at the car. Here, take my keys."

"Okay." Yolanda leaves the room.

"Daddy…"

"Yes, sweetie?"

"Why didn't I get my magic potion?"

"Your doctor believed that you weren't strong enough for it."

"But I am strong."

"I know you are, sweetie, but you did get some magic medicine to help with the meanies hurting you. Did it help?"

"Yeah, it did make the meanies go away."

"Good, sweetie."

"Daddy… why do you look sad?"

Michael just smiles. "Daddy isn't sad. I am just worried about you. That's all."

"Is there something you are not telling me, Daddy?"

"No, sweetie. It's just I am very worried about all of you soldiers, and each time you all come here I get very nervous." Michael strokes her hair. "I love you so much, sweetie."

Annabelle smiles. "I love you so much too, Daddy."

"Let's see if Daddy can get you out of here."

"Okay."

Michael calls the nurse in.

"Hi, Michael, is there something you need?"

"I was just wondering if I can take Annabelle home now."

"Yes, she is already discharged. You may take her home if you would like to."

"Thank you, nurse. I really do appreciate everything you all do here."

"Michael, it's no problem at all. Take care, Annabelle."

"Bye," Annabelle says, waving.

"Let's go, sweetie."

"Okay."

They then leave and meet everyone where they are waiting in the car.

"Let me help you in, sweetie."

"I got it, Daddy."

"Okay, sweetie."

Annabelle gets in her seat, Michael shuts the door and gets in the driver seat, and they head home.

"Hey, sissy, did you beat up the meanies with your magic potion?"

"I didn't get my magic potion today."

"You didn't? How come?"

"Buddy, she got some magic medicine to help her today."

"Oh, okay."

"Michael, why didn't she get her treatment?"

"Aunt Ruthie, it's because her doctor decided that all she needed was just magic medicine today."

"Uh huh, I see. Michael we shall discuss this later."

"I wouldn't have it any other way, Aunt Ruthie. Sweetie, I know that you are tired back there, but are you hungry?"

"I'm very tired, Daddy."

"I know, sweetie, but I really think you should eat something if you are up for it."

"I just want to go to bed, Daddy, if that's okay."

"Of course, sweetie."

They then arrive home and enter the house.

"Okay buddy, princess, you can have a little playtime to yourselves while we get situated here."

"Okay,." Gabriel says, running off.

"Aunt Ruthie, I know you spent today watching them, but do you think you can keep an eye on them for me?"

"Hush, Michael, these are my babies."

"Thank you, Aunt Ruthie. Yolanda, it's late enough as it is, do you mind doing me a favor?"

Yolanda smiles. "I will get dinner out, Michael. Just make sure my little cutie is okay."

"Thank you."

"What do you have in mind?"

"Chef's choice. You know what they can and can't have."

"Okay, Michael."

"Sweetie I know you are very tired, but I need you to get something in your tummy for your magic medicine. How about some fruit or yogurt?"

"Yogurt please."

"Okay sweetie. You may go to your room, and I will bring it to you."

"Okay."

"Can you go on your own?"

"Yes, Daddy, I can walk."

"I know that you are strong, sweetie. I just wanted to make sure."

"I know." She then goes into her room as Michael grabs a yogurt.

"Yolanda, I am going to be in Annabelle's room. If dinner is ready, go ahead and let everyone start without me."

"Okay Michael."

He then grabs Annabelle's medicines and goes to her room. "Hey sweetie, I know you are exhausted and are tired of people asking you this, but how are you feeling?"

"I am okay. Just very tired, and my tummy hurts a little."

"That is why you must eat so that I can give you this magic medicine to help you. Here is your yogurt."

"Thank you."

"You are very welcome."

She begins to eat slowly. "Daddy…"

"Yes sweetie?"

"Why did my doctor give me more medicine?"

"Well, Annabelle, it's because you couldn't get your magic potion, so she gave you this medicine to help fight the meanies."

"Daddy, remember I told you that I am a big girl?"

"I do, sweetie."

"You looked sad at Adventure Land, and you look sad now. What's wrong? Is it me?"

"You know I will never lie to you all, so I must tell you that after they took pictures of your heart, they noticed…"

"They noticed what, Daddy?"

Michael looking in her eyes could not tell her. "They noticed that your heart wasn't strong enough for magic potion today. That's all, sweetie."

"Is that why you look so sad?"

"I'm just very worried about all you soldiers. It's nothing for you to be worried about, sweetie."

"Why are we sick, Daddy?"

Michael, shocked by what she just asked, can only tell her, "Annabelle, I can't answer that. As much as it pains me, I don't have an honest answer for you. All I can tell you is to never give up fighting. God has his reasons so we must remain faithful and trust in our Father's plans. Remember to always have hope, faith, and love, as well, so that you may fight the meanies."

"I always do, Daddy. I'm done with my yogurt."

"Okay, sweetie, here is your little cup to help with the meanies so that you may sleep well tonight."

"Okay, thank you." She takes the medicine cup and drinks them with some juice.

"All gone, Daddy."

"Very good, sweetie. Are you up for a prayer?"

"Always, Daddy, but can you say one? My eyes keep wanting to shut."

"Of course I will, sweetie. You just drift into dreamland, but before you sleep, if you need anything at all, do not hesitate to call out for me or your aunts."

"Okay Daddy…" she says, closing her eyes as Michael softly speaks.

"Sweetheart, I know you are almost at dreamland, so I will say a prayer."

"Okay," she whispers.

"Dear Lord, our Father in heaven, please come down with your healing hand and touch this beautiful child of yours. Heal her from anything that is trying to harm her. Give her the strength to keep fighting on. In your heavenly name, Jesus, I pray. Amen."

Michael notices that she is sleeping and just stares for a moment, then softly whispers to her, "Sweetie, fight for me. Fight whatever is trying to get you. I know our Father is calling you home, but please stay here with me and fight. Our Father may need you, but sweetie," he tears up, "I need you." He then shuts the lights off and leaves the door open and makes his way to the dining room where everyone is sitting at the table.

"Just in time for everyone to finish, Michael. Where were you for so long?"

"Sorry about that. I was with Annabelle."

"This whole time?"

"Yes, Aunt Ruthie. I just wanted to make sure she was okay. You know how I get."

Aunt Ruthie sees that Michael is holding back something. "Uh huh."

"Anyways, Michael, your plate is covered for you."

"Thank you, Yolanda. This looks delicious."

"Oh, yeah it is, Daddy. It's yummy!"

"I'm glad you approve, buddy. To be honest, I don't have much of an appetite now, but thank you for cooking. Besides, it's way past time for medicines and their baths."

"Yolanda, just gave them their medicines and she volunteered to make sure they are ready for bed." You did Yolanda? "Yes, I in fact did." I appreciate that but I will get them ready for bed."

"No, Michael, you are going to sit here, and we are going to have a chat."

"Uh oh, someone is in trouble."

"Yeah, Daddy, you are in trouble," Gabriel says mockingly.

"Yolanda, please take these babies and make sure they are ready for bed."

"Yes ma'am."

"Give me hugs, soldiers."

"Okay."

"'Kay."

He hugs both Jazmyn and Gabriel. "I love you both so much. Goodnight."

"I love you too, Daddy. Night, night."

"Love you."

"Now, please remember to say your prayers."

"Okay."

"'Kay."

"Let's go, cuties." Yolanda takes Gabriel and Jazmyn in the back.

"I must clean up."

"No, you are not. You are going to sit here and tell me what is bothering you so much that it's basically written on your face."

"Aunt Ruthie, it's nothing. Really."

"Michael, you may be able to tell someone else that, but I know you and something is bothering you. Son, just tell me."

Michael knew that he couldn't say what was bothering him. "Aunt Ruthie, I don't know why God hasn't answered my prayers. My children are going through so much that now they are suffering from their illnesses. I just don't understand why this is happening."

"Look Michael, you know God works in mysterious ways. He has a reason for everything that goes on in this world. I am so very sorry that those babies of yours are sick, but don't lose your faith."

"I'm not, Aunt Ruthie, it's just that hasn't enough happened to us? It's bad enough they lost their mother and have these illnesses, but now they are suffering. I just don't understand how such a loving God will allow this to happen."

"Michael, you know our Father will never cause us pain. He loves us."

"Then if that is the case, why are they having pain?" Michael puts his head down. "Why am I in so much pain?"

"Michael, I know you must feel that way now, but you must understand everything that happens to us is according to His will."

"Forgive me, Aunt Ruthie, but is that why my children are on the verge of…"

"Of what, Michael?"

"I apologize. I just want to know what I can do to help my children. I want to know why at this very moment that I need Him—no, scratch that—my children need Him, He is nowhere to be found. I have always been and still am a faithful man, but it's just so hard to see my sweet, innocent children who have nothing but love for our Father suffer."

"Michael, it breaks my heart to hear you speak this way. You know for a fact that God loves us. There is nothing that I can say that will be comforting for you. I will tell you this, there is only one thing you can do."

"I know that, Aunt Ruthie, and believe me when I say that I pray all the time. I pray before I wake; before I sleep or eat; I even pray throughout the day. I think I pray so much that He has stopped listening."

"Michael, you don't honestly believe that. Do you?"

"Now, yes, I do."

"You can never pray enough. Michael, you are the most caring, loving, faithful man I know. You must not forget that. Everything will work out, Michael. Just believe."

"I do believe. I believe in our Father, in my children, and I believe in you and Yolanda."

"You are leaving someone out, Michael."

"Who?"

"You must believe in yourself, Michael. It's a good thing that you believe in everyone else, but you must first believe in yourself. That reminds me of something you had told us at dinner a while back. You said something that in order to love someone you must first what?"

Michael, trying to hold back a smile, says, "You must first love yourself."

"Exactly my point. Just as you told us, for love to blossom, it must first start with you. That works in any situation, Michael. Whether it's hope, faith, or love, you first must have those in yourself before giving it."

"I do have those, and I truly believe in what I say, but..."

"You must practice what you preach, Michael."

"Thank you, Aunt Ruthie."

"Any time that I am able to help, Michael. I am always here for you and those babies of yours."

"That means a lot to us."

Yolanda comes out. "Hey, what did I miss?"

"Nothing, Yolanda. Did they get to sleep okay?"

"Oh yes, they did. Right after their baths, they basically passed out on me."

"Yeah, that's their medicines. That is why right after they take their medicines, I send them for their baths."

"Noted for next time."

"Did you do a monster check for my little buddy?"

Yolanda laughs. "Yeah, although he was tired, he made me do one. Even though he said I didn't do it as good as you, he still went to bed."

Michael smiles. "Yeah, I should have warned you about that. You will get the hang of it. Did you also—"

Yolanda interrupts Michael. "Yes, they both said their prayers, Michael. I am beat. Those are my cuties, but boy do they wear you out."

Everyone smiles.

"Yes, that may be true, but we love them."

"You have that right. I am going to bed now."

"As am I. I hear my bed calling for me."

Michael gives both a hug. "I love you both so much, with all my heart. I truly am blessed to have both of you in my life. I wouldn't know what to do without you two. May you both have peaceful dreams tonight.

Aunt Ruthie, with smile, says, "I love you too, Michael, and for the record, though I can't speak for Yolanda, it is I who am blessed to be part of your family."

"I agree 100 percent with Aunt Ruthie, Michael. I love you too. You are not going to bed?"

"No, I think I just need to sit here and think for a while."

"About what?"

"I just need to connect with our Father again."

"See, that's the kind of thing I want to come out of your mouth Michael."

"Thank you again, Aunt Ruthie, Yolanda."

"For what?" they both say, puzzled as Michael smiles.

"For everything you both do for us and for reminding me that I need a life preserver on my journey."

Yolanda and Aunt Ruthie both smile.

"You're welcome, Michael. Goodnight."

"Goodnight, Michael."

"Goodnight, ladies."

"Get some rest, Michael."

"I will, Yolanda."

Yolanda and Aunt Ruthie go into their rooms to retire for the night, and Michael goes into the dark living room, sits in his chair, and says a prayer.

"Father, Lord, if you can still hear me, I, once again, ask of you to please save and heal my children. I'm lost in this world, Lord, and I don't know where to turn. I ask and ask of you for guidance, but I have yet to hear from you. I know in my heart that you are everywhere, guiding and watching over us, but it just feels like you have abandoned us. Forgive me, Father, for what is in my heart, but these are my children. In fact, Lord, they are your children. Why must they go through this? Why put such loving children through so much torment?"

Michael, filled with emotion, fights his tears. "Why must you put me through so much pain? Father, I pray unto you to tell me what I must do to heal them." Michael's tears begin to fall. "Lord, what must I do to save my children? I will never try to bargain with you, Lord, but please, tell me what I must do. Take me, Lord, not my innocent children."

Michael begins to cry. "Please, God, don't take my children from me."

As Michael sits in his chair, he hears a noise.

Chapter 9

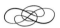

"Yolanda? Aunt Ruthie? Soldiers? Hello?" Michael hears nothing but silence and jumps up in a panic. "Who is out here?"

He then hears a voice behind him. "Hello, Michael."

Michael, startled, begins to speak in a firm voice. "What?! I don't know how you got past the alarm, but just take whatever it is that you want and please leave. I won't call the police, just leave!"

The once-dark room is filled with light.

"Michael, do not be frightened."

"Who are you?"

"I am a messenger from above."

"From where and from whom?"

"From God, Michael."

"This cannot be true. I must have fallen asleep and now I am dreaming," Michael says, trying to rationalize the situation. "Yes, I am dreaming."

"No, Michael, you are not dreaming."

"What are you?"

"We have many names, but you may be familiar with the most common. I am an angel, Michael."

"An angel?"

"Yes, an angel, Michael."

"This cannot be happening because I know an angel doesn't just come down to talk with us. Especially one sent from God."

"Do you know that, Michael?"

"Well yes, I do."

"You have faith, right?"

"Of course I do."

"Although you can't see or hear heaven, you believe it's there, right?"

"Yes…"

"You also believe in a divine power that created and watches over this world, right?"

"Well yes, I do."

"Then you know that I am here in front of you with a message from our Father."

"What is your name?"

The angel chuckles. "You humans and always needing a name. For the sake of argument, just call me Angel."

"Wait this can't be real, but okay Angel. What are you doing here?"

"As I said Michael, I have a message from God."

"You are not here to take my children, are you?"

"Let's discuss that. Please have a seat, Michael."

"You can't take my children. There is no way I can allow that."

"Michael, if our Father sees fit, he will call anyone he pleases to return home. Now, please sit so that we may discuss some things."

Michael, still in shock, can only say, "Okay, I will."

Michael and the angel sit down.

"There. Isn't that better, Michael?"

"What do you need to tell me about my children? I know that is why you are here."

"You have asked our Father on many occasions what you can do to heal and save your children."

"Okay…"

"I am here to tell you that our Father has answered your prayers."

"Great! So, when is this going to happen?"

"We will get to that soon, Michael, but first let's have a discussion."

"What is there to discuss? All I care about is my children's wellbeing."

The angel smiles. "I know you do, but don't you have any questions for me?"

"Not really, no."

"Michael, not only are you talking to an angel but one who is sent from God. I know that you are still trying to wrap your head around if this is real or not, but I assure you that this real. You must have many questions for me. So here I am. Go ahead ask me anything you would like."

Michael could only think of one question at that moment. "Why was Anna taken from us?"

"I figured that would be your first question."

"Please tell me. Why did my children lose their mother and why did I lose my wife?"

"Michael, Anna's purpose in life was fulfilled."

"How can that be? She had a family!"

"Michael, please lower your voice. You don't want your family to come out here and see you talking to yourself because I am only here for you."

Michael begins to speak in a normal tone. "Anna had a lot more to see. Jazmyn's first steps, our children's birthdays, Christmases, our anniversaries. She… she just had so much life left to live and now she is gone."

"Michael, do you honestly believe Anna left you all? She may not be here in the physical sense, but look what she did for you. You yourself were on a dark path. Your faith was being tested every day, then what happened?"

"What?"

"Michael, Anna had showed you power that you have never seen before, that no other can take from you. She showed you love, Michael, and you know this to be true."

"I understand that, but why isn't she here now?"

"It was her time, Michael. Anna did everything God had asked of her to do."

"What do you mean by that?"

"To start, Anna birthed a family. She instilled love and faith unto you all and tasked you to carry that on. That was her purpose in life, and you are doing a great job of doing so. For the record, your sister and aunt were right when they said that heaven is smiling upon you because of the way you are raising your children and the way you treat everyone around you, because we are."

"I just miss her so much."

"I know that you do, Michael, but you must understand; when a purpose is fulfilled in life, it's time to return home."

"I do understand that. I must ask this, why do my children have not just cancers but rare cancers? All of them. Why would a loving God give them such illnesses and not let them be normal children?"

"Michael, what is your definition of normal?"

"Off the top of my head, someone who can do normal activities."

"Is a person not normal if they don't have an arm? A leg? Is a person not normal if they are confined to a wheelchair? A bed?"

"That's not fair because you know I don't see the disabled or handicapped as abnormal."

"My point, Michael, is that you humans all look at the wrong picture, judging what is normal or isn't normal. You all here see what you want to see. I will help you out to see it more clearly. Say there is a person out in this world, and this person is someone who believes in themselves no matter what is going on in life, whether life has been good to this person or not, he or she still goes through life with nothing but love in his or her heart and a smile on his or her face. Now allow me to ask you this, would that person not be considered normal?"

"I see your point, but what about those who are homeless? Children all over the world who go hungry—mothers, fathers everywhere who can't provide for their families. What do you call that?"

"I would call it an opportunity."

"An opportunity? For what?"

"An opportunity for you all to help one another. An opportunity to believe in yourselves. To believe in our Father. Surely our Father can snap his fingers and end it all, but at what cost?"

"I don't follow."

"You see, you all expect miracles to suddenly appear and end things that you yourselves can end. You all perform miracles every day by helping one another. We see it more often than you might think. When you see someone starving, you feed them. When you see someone that needs assistance, you help them. If there are those who are without clothes, you give them yours. You see, you all here on Earth might think that those are just little gestures to help your fellow brother and sister, but to that person one little act of random kindness will get them through their tough times. How can our Father take that away from you all? If our Father were to snap his fingers and make everything go away, how can any of you know the power of love and what joy those things doing brings to someone?"

"What about those suffering in the world?"

"What is suffering, Michael?"

"That's easy, it's someone who is going through so much turmoil in their lives and has nowhere to turn."

"You call that suffering, Michael?"

"Well yes, I do. That is basically the definition of suffering."

"Michael, once again you are mistaken."

"What do you call it then?"

"I see someone who is what you call suffering as someone who never gives up. Someone who has faith and trusts in our Father will never go without."

"There are plenty of people who have faith and trust in the Lord but still go without food and shelter every day. It breaks my heart."

"Michael, are there not food assistance programs throughout this world? Are there not shelters in place to help those in need who search for it? There are many programs to help those who are suffering by your definition."

"Well yes, there are, but I am curious what you will call someone who is suffering. Give me your definition of suffering."

"I will call those who are suffering are ones who have given up on the world. Those who have given up on themselves and those who have given up on our Father. Those who blame everyone around them and blame our Father for everything that is happening to them. Some people seem to forget that, although you all were given free will, for every bad decision or action, there must be consequences. That right there, Michael, is my definition of suffering."

"It just does not make sense to me."

"What are you confused about, Michael?"

"We are all God's children, right?"

"Yes."

"Then look at the world and the state that we are in."

"Exactly, Michael, look at it."

"Wait, now I am even more confused."

"Tell me, Michael, when you look at the world what do you see?"

"I see wars going on; I see hospitals being filled more and more every day; I see children being diagnosed with illnesses and many that are diagnosed terminal." Michael puts his head down. "I see my children's futures slimming every day. Why would such a loving God allow all this happen to his children if he loves us so much? I just do not understand it."

"Michael, and as God's children do you think our Father will abandon you all? Will you as a Father abandon your children?"

"You know I will never abandon my children on any circumstance."

"Neither will our Father. He has a plan and reason for everything that goes on in this world."

"Now you sound like my aunt."

"Good and you should listen to her because she is correct. You all must have faith and believe in our Father. You all must put your trust in our Father."

"I do. It's just very hard, and it feels like we are alone sometimes, especially now with what is going on with my children."

"Faith and trust are never easy, Michael. If it were, then everyone would have it. Faith and trust must be fought for and earned. You are a living testimony of that."

"I understand that, but it still feels like God just stopped loving us; like our Father just gave up on the world."

"Never, Michael, will our Father ever give up on you all. Since the time of your creation, He has loved you all and always will. What you all here on Earth fail to see is that God loves you all so much that he gave you all His only son. To put it as in your metaphor, our Father gave you all a life preserver."

Michael smiles. "How do you know about that?"

The angel just gives Michael a look. "We know everything, Michael, and our Father is very pleased with you. Especially with your definitions, stories, and metaphors. We all just love hearing them."

"That is very comforting to hear, but it still doesn't explain why, if He loves us so much, we are all in such turmoil."

"Michael, our Father loves you all so much that he wants you all home with us in our Father's kingdom. That is why he gave you all a wonderful gift, his son, your Lord and Savior, Jesus Christ."

"And look what we did with that gift."

"You all are misinformed on that subject and misinterpret the message."

"I beg you to please enlighten me and tell me what we are missing."

"Our Father saw what this world as it stood and had seen something must be done to help you all. So, He gave the world a chance by giving you all His son. Jesus saw the world and where you all were heading so in order to be your savior, He did the only thing He knew that was going to save you all. Jesus loves you all so much that he gave you all himself on the cross on that day. Surely all of heaven was ready on the word of Jesus to come down and stop it, but with his dying breath he asked our Father to forgive you all for you not know what you are doing. That is the amazing thing about love. Jesus knew by sacrificing himself for you all on the cross that you all will have a fighting chance."

"A fighting chance for what?"

"A chance to come home, Michael."

"But look at us. Look at the news. How can we all honestly think that we are worthy of entering the kingdom of heaven?"

"One simple reason, Michael, because of the blood shed on the cross that day, a door was opened to you all. Always remember that no one may enter the kingdom of heaven without Jesus. He is the way to our Father, and no one may go to our Father but through Jesus Christ. Unfortunately, there are many that forget that you all were given a wonderful gift of forgiveness. Some take that for granted. There are many that live by their own rules, and yes, many don't believe in our Father, but he loves everyone just as much. God and Jesus will never stop loving you all. Our Father and your Lord and Savior believe in you all so much that they are waiting for you all to come home. All of you may enter the kingdom of heaven only if you believe in our Father and accept Jesus Christ in your hearts as your Lord and Savior. Do you understand now, Michael?"

"I do. I am just having trouble comprehending something."

"What is troubling you, Michael?"

"I understand how loved we are, and I know how powerful love is…"

"Just say what is on your mind, Michael."

"It just doesn't seem right that our Father, who does in fact love us, would give my children these types of illnesses. What did they do to deserve this kind of life? What did I do in my life that was so bad that Anna was taken from not only me but from them as well? Why put them such through a horrible life? What I am trying to say is why would God allow them such a life?"

"What exactly kind of life do they have, Michael?"

"Well, their treatments, doctors, having to go to the hospital every day, and now…" Michael sheds a tear. "Come Monday, it looks to be like no life at all. I just do not understand it."

"Michael, you are looking at it differently than what your eyes can see."

Michael wipes away his tears. "Please explain it to me because I am lost. What am I missing?"

"Your children are loved deeply by both of their fathers. By our Father above and by you down here on Earth. Your children experience what many do not get to experience in their lifetime."

"What's that?"

"Your children know the true meaning of happiness."

"Happiness?" Michael says, confused.

"Yes, Michael happiness. They have a father who loves them so much and will do whatever it takes for them to smile. Am I correct?"

"Well yes, you are, but it is my job to make them smile."

"No Michael. That is your love for them. You love your family so much that your love is more powerful than you can ever imagine."

"How so?"

"For the simple fact that you don't tell them they are going to a hospital. Where do you tell them they are going for treatments and visits?"

"Adventure land."

"Exactly Michael. You created a world for your children to be as one. You created this world within yourselves so that they may have something to experience in like a theme park. You really do not understand what you did, do you?"

"No, I just created adventure land because they were scared, and I wanted them to feel safe and turn something that terrifies most children, even parents, into a fun adventure. That is all I did to be honest with you."

"Michael, you did more than that. Your children only have hope because you created it for them. They have faith because you show them every day what the true meaning of faith is. Your children feel the power of love, because you refuse to show them anything less than that. Michael, that is the true definition of happiness. Your children get to experience these things because of you. Many go through their life in search of just one of those traits—your children have all three. Michael, what do you think about that? I will call that a miracle, and it's the love from you that did that. If I am wrong, then you tell me what you would call that."

"No, you are right—it is a miracle. I just don't know if I can carry on any further than where I am at. I need strength."

The angel smiles. "Michael, I can get up and show you where your strength is, but I don't really need to do that, do I?"

"What do you mean?"

"You have strength in those three beautiful children sleeping in their beds. You have strength in your sister and aunt. You have strength all around you. They are truly blessed as are you."

"Forgive me but how so?"

"Yes, your children have these illnesses, but they go in for their treatments, or shall I say magic potions, with hope that they are going to be better. They have faith in our Father that everything is going to be okay. Your children have love in their hearts, because they know that they are cared for. Your children are very strong, Michael. Where do you think they get their strength from?"

"I don't know, but I tell you this—don't tell them that they aren't going to beat their illnesses, because they don't know the definition of giving up."

"Your children have strength because you give it to them, Michael. It comes from you. You and your family are the definition of strength. You do not need strength, Michael, because it's right here in your family."

"You know I meet and hear people every day say, 'oh I am sorry for what you are going through' or 'what can I do to help.' Although I appreciate the sentiment, I sometimes feel they say that because they feel sorry for my children.

"And don't you feel sorry for those people?"

"I do, because those kinds of people don't understand my children, and children in hospitals everywhere don't need people to feel sorry for them. They just need people to understand how tough they are fighting these illnesses—what they are going through. They just need people to believe in them as they do. It breaks my heart to see people that don't understand these things and continue to treat them as if they are gone."

"Michael, then teach those that do not understand. Show them, so that they may understand it."

"I try all the time, but it seems like they aren't ready to."

"Then prepare them on how to be ready, Michael." "

"I will try harder, but I feel like my children are somehow being punished."

"How did you come to that conclusion, Michael?"

"I don't know. Maybe I didn't pray enough, go to church as often as I should have, or maybe I just wasn't Christian enough. The angel laughs.

"Michael, why do you say that you are not Christian enough?"

"Honestly, I don't know why I said that."

"Michael, what does not being Christian enough mean to you?"

"I don't know, maybe not reading the bible as much as I should have."

"Okay, Michael, here is your chance to show me how Christian you are."

"How do I do that?"

"I hate to point out the irony in this, but you are having a conversation with an angel, Michael, and you still say that you are not Christian enough. Here is your chance to prove to me how Christian you are."

"How do you propose I do that?"

"Quickly, off the top of your head, tell me a bible verse, any verse, and not John 3:16 either."

"I am mad at myself for saying this to an angel, but I can't now."

"You can't?"

"Not off the top of my head, no."

"Exactly my point, Michael."

"What?"

"You all wonder around this Earth, spending your lifetimes in searching and judging what and who is good enough for our Father. Many of you miss the whole point."

"Isn't that how it is supposed to be?"

"No, Michael."

"Then how will we know if we are good enough for our Father?"

"He who believes in me shall not perish but in turn have everlasting life. I am pretty sure you have heard of that before, right?"

"Well of course I have, and I do believe. That is not problem."

"Then what is the problem, Michael?"

"It's just I don't know what more I can do."

"Believe in yourself, Michael. It's that simple. Your children certainly believe in you. As does our Father, Lord, and Savior. All the Lord asks of you all is to believe in him and know that you will have everlasting life in the kingdom of heaven."

"I understand that, but how does this apply to my children? They certainly believe in our Father and accept Jesus as their Lord and Savior in their hearts."

"Michael, it has everything to do with your children."

"How so?"

"They believe not because you told them that they must believe but because you believe, Michael. You can't make someone believe. Let me ask you this: Do you believe our Father created this world and put you all down here to bow down to him like a dictator?"

"No, of course not."

"Exactly Michael. Our Father gave you all free will but, as I said to you before, a door was opened to you all with a key. The only way you may enter is to accept Jesus as your Lord and Savior and, through Jesus, our Father will welcome you all home with open arms, but you all must believe and trust him to come home. Whether you believe or not with free will, it's up to you all if you want everlasting life or not. I will say this: Our Father certainly believes in you all."

"I know you said our Father had sent you to speak to me about my children and something about my prayers being answered. Although I know this is maybe a once-in-a-lifetime opportunity to speak with you, please tell me about my children. What must I do to heal and save my children? I will do anything. I certainly have faith in our Father, and I know that he has a plan for us all, but what must I do for my children?"

"You are right about one thing: Our Father does have a plan in place for you all."

"Please tell me what it is."

"Yes, the reason I was sent to speak with you is not to talk about everything we had discussed but about your children—that is why I am here."

"What is it?"

"You have prayed repeatedly about what you must do to heal and save your children, and, as I said earlier, our Father has sent me to give you a message.

I am here to tell you, just as He always does, He is listening and has heard your cries and has answered your prayers." Michael gets up from excitement.

"Okay, great! When can they stop going to the hospital? When can they stop getting their treatments? When can they play outside? When can they go to school?"

"I am only a messenger. Please sit down." Michael begins to sit back down but notices the angel's voice change.

"Okay... but why are you talking that way?"

"Your children will be healed from their illnesses under one condition."

"Okay, great! Anything! Just tell me it's done!"

"Not so fast, Michael."

"What is the condition?"

"This is what our Father is asking of you, Michael." Michael can't take anymore suspense.

"Please tell me."

"Michael in order for them to be healed... I am sorry to tell you this, but one must come home." Michael is shocked by what he just heard from the angel.

"What?! What do you mean one must go home?"

"Our Father is tasking you with a decision, Michael. You must decide which of your child goes home to heal the other two."

"What?! I cannot just decide which child goes home to heal the other two! How can this be?! I... No! There is no way that I can do that!"

"Michael, this is our Father's will. This is what He is asking of you to do."

"No! I will not decide on which of my children goes home! This is their home! How can such a loving God do this?!"

"That is the point, Michael. Our Father is loving. This is what our Father is asking of you to do. It is for you to decide. I am sorry, and I wish there were another way, but this is what needs to be done in order to heal your children."

"No!"

"Michael, as you and I both know, thy will be done."

"But please go talk to Him. Please tell Him there must be another way to heal my children! Please."

"I am sorry, but it is said. Michael, at midnight on Sunday I will be back for you to tell me your decision and Michael please try to understand, this is what needs to be done." Or what?! What if I don't decide let's call it what it is, sacrifice one of my children, then what?!

"If you don't decide, then I am afraid that I will come back three times to bring them all home. Michael, please obey our Father's command. This your task. Decide wisely, as I may only come once at midnight."

"How can you, an angel, sit there and tell me to give you one of them?! Go look at them! How can you tell me that at midnight one of my sweet innocent children is going home?!" Michael, in shock and full of emotions, begins to realize what must happen and softly asks the angel, "How can this be?"

"Michael I am only a messenger of God. This how our Father is answering your prayers. This, I am afraid, is what will happen with or without your decision. You can decide on one to return home or all three. That is your decision to make. So, go forth and cherish your time with your children. Do not lose your faith in our Father, for He will never lose faith in you.

Always remember that our Father will never give you more than you can handle."

"What do I do?"

"Love one another as you always do, Michael. Never lose your love for our Father, for He will never stop loving you. Never lose hope in our Father, because this is the way to heal your children, for He has hope in you that you will obey this command and decide."

"I just can't decide... it's too much! They are my children! They are the reason why my love for our Father is so strong! And now you are telling me I must decide... No! This cannot be..." Michael succumbs to his emotions. "What if I just..." The angel interrupts.

"No Michael, I am afraid not. This is our Father's will. Again, Michael, decide wisely, and the others shall be healed."

"So, you are telling me that I have two days left with one of my children! Or that my other option is that, if I don't decide, I lose all three?! What kind of God is that?!"

"A loving God, Michael. Our Father loves you all so much that there is a home waiting in his kingdom for all of you. Just think, Michael—no more treatments for your children. No more doctors, hospitals. No more praying for a miracle, because this is your miracle, Michael, and our Father is tasking you to give it. Our Father has made this promise to you: Come Monday, your children will be able to go outside and play. Just think about that. No more pain. No more sleepiness nights. No more medicines, because you are giving your children the ultimate medicine directly from our Father. Can you imagine the possibilities?"

"I can, but I just don't know if my faith will be able to withstand this decision."

"Michael, your faith is what brought you here to this very moment. Please do not lose your faith. Have faith and trust in our Father. He is giving you this decision not to punish you in any way but to give you a once-in-a-lifetime opportunity."

"What's that? Sacrifice one of my children?"

"No Michael our Father is giving you an insight in His plans. Isn't that what you wanted all along? Isn't that what you had prayed for?"

"Yes, I did, but not like this. Does our Father's plan include me resenting him?"

"No Michael."

"How can you ask a man who already lost his wife to give up one of his children? Or all of them at that? How? Or is this a test? Am I Abraham and, suddenly, our Father will at the last minute send you down to tell me that our Father was just testing me to see if I obeyed? Please tell me that is what is happening here." The angel smiles at Michael.

"So, you do know the bible."

"I told you I didn't off the top of my head."

"Listen to the words you are saying Michael."

"What words are those?"

"Resent, take, tests…Michael, our Father does not play games with you, and He didn't take anything from you."

"I beg to differ! He took my wife! My love! My children's mother!"

"She went home because, as I explained to you, it was her time. Let me ask this of you. Do you believe in love?"

"Yes, I do because she was it! I can never love anything or anyone as much as I loved her!"

"What about your children?"

"That is not fair! You know I love them more than I love myself! More than anything in this world!"

"How did you come about the love for them?"

"I… I just can't explain it."

"Try to, Michael."

"As I held each one of my children when they were born, nothing else mattered in this world but to show them what love is. It was almost the same love that I had for Anna but more. I can't explain it."

"Exactly, Michael. Our Father loves you so much that He created Anna just for you."

"I always felt that way, but I must ask you, why?"

"As I told you earlier, you were headed on a dark path. You were going to be the definition of suffering. You honestly do not see that, do you?"

"No, but to be honest with you, I feel like I am suffering now with what you said I must do."

"Michael, you know that is not what I am asking you."

"Okay, but about love—I know that when I met Anna, I had never felt that strong about anything in my life. Then when my children were born, I knew love on another level. A type of love that I have never experienced before in my life."

"That's my point Michael."

"What is?"

"You were gifted of the power of love. An emotion that you never felt before. The love you have feel for your children is the same love that our Father has you for you all. It's the same love that Jesus has for all of humanity. The love in heaven for you all is greater than your minds can ever imagine. I told you earlier our Father can easily snap his fingers, and all of humanity's problems will go away, but will come of that?"

"Well to start there will be no more diseases, no more hate in the world, there will be no more pain."

"Then we will all be in heaven wouldn't we?"

"Yes."

"Michael, you all fail to see the opportunities in each other. How can humanity ever experience true friendship, true love?"

"I am trying to understand you, but I can't."

"Say there is a mother or father who has all the money in the world and showers their child or children with everything that they ask for. Is that love?"

"Well no."

"Why isn't that love?"

"Because you can't buy love."

"Say there is a businesswoman with endless connections. Does she ever experience true friendship?"

"Well no, she does not."

"Why not?"

"Because those that want to get close will only want her for her connections."

"A parent who wakes up early everyday regardless of what shift he or she works just to make their child's favorite meal. One who works sixty-hour work weeks just to provide a roof over their family's heads and keeps food on the table, A parent who works overtime just to provide birthdays, Thanksgiving, Christmas, just to see their family smile. Is that love?"

"Of course it is."

"Tell me why?"

"For the simple fact that anyone that loves their family that much to do all that has to be driven by love."

"Very good. Let's say there is a person that has someone they can call no matter what time it is and drop everything they are doing for each other to be with them during the good and bad times. Is that true friendship?"

"Yes of course."

"Why is that?"

"Because it is in the same category of love, and they care for one another, but you said money isn't the key. What about those parents who are out of work? Those that are alone in this world? Those without homes?"

"You are missing the point, Michael."

"Can you please help me understand what is the point?"

"The point of these examples is that many go through life with nothing but hope that everything will be better. They have faith in our Father that He will provide for them. They have love for one another. You see, Michael, with those traits those people will never go without."

"Forgive me for saying this, but does our Father's plan consist of bad things happening to good people so that we will turn to our Father and ask Him for help?"

"No Michael. Free will, remember? Our Father cannot make you do that. As I told you, our Father cannot make you put your trust in Him, to love Him, to believe in Him. That is something you all must do on your own. Yes, there are many that are lost, those that do evil deeds, but you must understand our Father is a forgiving God."

"I am truly sorry, but what about my children? How does all this apply to them?"

"Michael this is your chance."

"For?"

"A cross is being put up. It's up to you to decide who will bear that cross. You have free will and can either obey or disobey our Father, but remember that there are consequences for every bad decision and action. That is all the time I have for you until we meet again, but you must understand that you are not alone. You must understand that your children are not alone. There is a home waiting in heaven for whoever you decide. Michael, this is your sole purpose in life. Just know that you all will be reunited and live as one in the kingdom of heaven. This your task, Michael, so please decide wisely. Our Father believes that you will fulfill your destiny. For I will come at midnight on Sunday, and I will need your decision at that time."

"How will I know?"

"You will know, Michael. Your decision will be handed to you in such a manner that you will know when it is time. Goodbye, Michael." Just like that the angel leaves, and so does the light. Once again, Michael sits in the dark.

"What am I going to do?"

Chapter 10

Michael awakens to his alarm clock from his phone.

"Wow six in the morning already? Of course, I didn't get much rest. How could I after last night…or was it this morning? How am I supposed to decide something like this?" Michael tries to rationalize the situation.

"Maybe it was just a dream, but I don't even remember sleeping… or did I? Regardless if I slept or not, I must go check on my soldiers." He then gets up and goes to Jazmyn's room first, where of course she was wide awake.

"Daddy!!"

"Shh princess, we don't want to wake everyone else up at this hour. How is your bubble?"

"Ouchy."

"I am sorry princess. Let's get some food in your tummy so that you may take some medicine for the meanies to go away."

"K."

"Let's go in the kitchen princess." They both go out to the kitchen.

"Okay princess, do you want eggs or fruit?"

"Egg."

"Okay princess, coming right up." As he goes to prepare breakfast, he hears some noise and looks at Jazmyn. "Uh oh princess. I hear noise but it's way too early. I wonder who is up at this hour? Let's see who is up this early." They both look at the hallway in anticipation of seeing who is up, then out comes Annabelle and Gabriel.

"Daddy!!"

"Shh soldiers. We don't want to wake up your aunts. Hi soldiers. Good morning. What are you both doing up so early?"

"I had a good night's sleep, and I woke up feeling better."

"Me too, Daddy."

"I am glad to hear that soldiers. How are you two feeling?"

"Much better, those magic medicines really worked."

"I feel better too, Daddy. I don't have to poop that much." Michael smiles.

"That is very good news, soldiers. I am getting breakfast ready so you both may go and do what you feel."

"Okay" Gabriel runs into the living room.

"Toons!" Jazmyn shouts as she runs behind Gabriel.

"Yes princess, you may watch your cartoons. Buddy, will you please put cartoons on for your sister?"

"I already am."

"Thank you buddy."

"You're welcome. Here you go, Jazzy. Cartoons."

"Yay."

"Sweetie, you may go if you would like to or you can stay here. I don't mind."

"No imma go in a minute. Daddy…"

"Yes sweetie?"

"Where did you sleep last night?"

"I fell asleep on my chair in the living room… or at least I think I did. Why do you ask?"

"I woke up in the middle of the night, and I thought I heard you talking to someone. I was going to come out, but I fell back asleep." Michael at that moment realized what in fact occurred last night was validated.

"I may have been talking in my sleep, sweetie. It's nothing to worry about."

"Oh, okay. I do that sometimes, too."

"How do you know you are talking in your sleep if you are sleeping?"

"Because I have these amazing dreams, and I wake up like I am talking to someone that is right there in my room, but I know that it's a dream, so I go back to sleep."

"What are these amazing dreams?"

"Sometimes I am in this amazing place that is so beautiful that I can't describe it. I even have dreams that I am with Mommy." Gabriel overhears Annabelle.

"I have dreams like that. I dream about Mommy all the time too, Daddy!" Michael is puzzled.

"So, both of you dream of this amazing place and Mommy often?"

"Yup!" Gabriel shouted as he continued to watch television. "I do all the time."

"Sweetie, let me ask you this: How do you feel when you visit this place?"

"I feel safe, Daddy. Like nobody will ever hurt me, and I feel so much love, like I do for my family." Michael realizes what place they may be speaking of and tries hard not to react in a way to scare his children.

"That's good, sweetie. I am glad that you are having sweet dreams."

"Me too. I hate the meanie dreams."

"What are those?"

"Where meanies are alive and are chasing me, but then I pray, and they go away."

"You pray in your dream?"

"Yup. I sure do."

"I will be honest sweetie. I don't really know how to comment on that but to say that I am so glad you have the power to pray in your dreams."

"Me too."

"Who told you to pray in your dreams?"

"This man."

"Who?"

"I don't know. I never see his face, but I always feel safe when I hear him."

"Well sweetie, I am so glad to know that you are protected in your dreams."

"Me too. I am going to go in the living room now."

"Okay sweetie." Michael stood there in the kitchen wondering who they were talking to in their dreams, and he could only come up with one answer.

"Lord, I thank you for protecting my children not just in our world but in their dreams as well." Michael finishes cooking.

"Okay soldiers. Come and get it while it's hot!"

"Yes!" Gabriel comes running. "Already daddy? I didn't get to watch my video."

"I know sweetie, it's my fault for holding you up, but please come and sit at the table." Princess comes running to Michael and holds up her arms. "Up Daddy."

"Okay princess up you go. Let me just lock in your tray… and there you are. Now you are all set to eat. Here is your plate."

"Yay. Egg!" Michael smiles and serves Annabelle and Gabriel.

"Okay. We have your meals, drinks, what are we forgetting soldiers?"

"Grace!" Annabelle and Gabriel shout.

"Very good soldiers. Who wants to volunteer?"

"I will Daddy."

"Okay sweetie. You may begin when you're ready."

"We thank you Lord for this delicious meal you have blessed us with, and I thank you for making the meanies stop hurting us so that we can have a good day today. In Jesus's name we pray."

"Amen." Everyone says together.

"Very good sweetie. Everyone, go ahead and eat."

"Yes!" Gabriel says, grabbing his plate. "Daddy are you going to tell us a story today?"

"I was thinking we all enjoy each other's company and talk about some things."

"Like what?"

"Well sweetie, I know we went over what you both can and can't watch on your tablets and on television, but I was wondering something. When you watch your videos, are there any boys on there that you like?"

"Daddy! I'm not going to tell you that!" Michael laughs.

"Okay, okay. I understand you don't want to tell me, but I must tell you this. You will meet a lot of boys in your lifetime, and although many will come and go, someone very special will come along. You two will love each other so much that he will ask for your hand in marriage."

"How will I know if he is special?"

"How he shows his worthiness to you."

"Huh?"

"He will only be worthy for your hand if he treats you like the queen you will become."

"I become?"

"Yes, sweetie. As you know how I call Jazzy princess…"

"I princess!" Jazmyn interrupts.

"Yes, you are daddy's princess. Annabelle, no matter how old you are, you will always be my princess as well. A person that is worthy of you will take the princess that you are and treats you like his queen that you are destined to be."

"But how will I know?"

"Trust me sweetie, you will know in heart when the time comes."

"Like how?"

"Well, to start he will love you unconditionally and put you above himself. Someone who does whatever it takes to make you smile and keep that beautiful smile of yours on our face. If I had it my way, he would be a God-loving man, but that's just me. Anyways, as I was saying. Someone who is a true gentleman."

"I'm a gentleman Daddy."

"I know you are buddy, and I am very proud of you, but we are talking about your sister here."

"Oh yea."

"Sweetie, it's someone who opens the door for you. "

"Nobody does that Daddy. Only you do."

"Exactly sweetie. That is when you know you have true gentleman. Don't get me wrong, I am not sitting here calling myself a gentleman, because it's not something you can just call yourself. You must do the actions to prove it."

"You're one Daddy, because you always open the doors for us and say ladies first."

"Yes sweetie, I do but I am speaking of this special someone that you one day will meet. You are deeply loved by your family and heaven up above. Annabelle, when he can do those things for you and show you true love, he will be worthy to have you as his queen."

"I love you Daddy."

"I love you too Daddy."

"Love you." Michael smiles.

"I love you all so much."

"Daddy?"

"Yes sweetie."

"I have been dropping hints about my birthday, but we never talk about it. What are we doing for my birthday?" At that moment, everything that may come hits Michael.

"Daddy, are you okay?"

"You look like you seen the bogeyman."

"I'm sorry soldiers, Daddy was just thinking about something."

"Like what?"

"Nothing buddy." Michael looked at his children, faced with the reality of what the angel had told him.

"Soldiers. I know we went over this but give me an honest answer. How are you all feeling today?"

"I feel great!" Gabriel shouted.

"Princess?"

"I princess!"

"That answers that. And you sweetie?"

"I feel a lot better today. Why? What do you want to do today Daddy?"

"Well sweetie, I was thinking of having a genie day for my soldiers."

"Genie day?"

"What's that Daddy?"

"Well soldiers, we are going to pretend that I am a genie, and I am here to grant each of you soldiers a wish. We are going to do whatever your hearts desire today."

"Yay!!" The children shouted.

"Oh Daddy I want to play video games. No, I want to play laser tag! No wait! I want to ride cars!" Gabriel said with excitement.

"Okay buddy I hear you. Annabelle, what would you like to do?"

"I really want to go see where they make videos like on my tablet! I want to be in one! Can I Daddy?"

"Of course, sweetie. Anything for my soldiers. Princess, I know you will just come along for the ride, but we are going to do something special for you as well." Jazmyn giggles.

"Okay soldiers, with all that information, I know just the place to take you all."

"Where Daddy?"

"Please tell us Daddy!"

"It is a surprise! It's a good thing that you soldiers are finished eating your breakfast or else you all will just want to go get ready."

"Can we Daddy?!"

"In a minute buddy. First, you must line up for your medicines. Annabelle, here is your cup."

"Thank you."

"You're welcome. Gabriel, here is yours."

"Thank you, Daddy."

"Your welcome buddy. And princess, here is yours."

"K."

"You're welcome princess."

"All gone."

"Mine too."

"Gone"

"Wow soldiers! You all must be excited."

"I am."

"Me too."

"Okay solders, you may go get dressed so that we can leave soon, because I want to get there early so you all can do as you wished."

"Yay!!" The children shouted, hurrying to their rooms. At that moment, Yolanda came out due to all the commotion.

"Michael, what's going on and why are the cuties so excited?"

"Good morning to you too, sis."

"Good morning, Michael."

"I am sort of sorry they woke you, but I am glad they did. I told them today was genie day and, before you ask, I granted them wishes on whatever it is that they want to do today. With what they wished for, I know the perfect place."

"Where are you taking them?"

"They don't know this yet but we, as in all of us as a family, are going to The Land of Dreams."

"Land of Dreams? Where did that come from?"

"I think it's about time they get to experience what it feels like to be kids without all the doctors and hospitals. Yes, we have adventure land, but I think it's time to take them to a real theme park so that they may be children for once."

"Are you sure, Michael?"

"I have never been surer in my life than this, Yolanda. I just need you to trust me and I will need your help. Please."

"Of course, Michael, I will help you. You know I'm here for you all."

"Thank you so much Yolanda. I need this to go well for them. If you don't mind before or after you get dressed, can you get princess ready?"

"No problem Michael."

"Thank you again, Yolanda. I am going to wake Aunt Ruthie up, get ready, then I must get their bags packed with their medicines and extra clothes."

"Okay Michael. Let's go cutie." Yolanda takes Jazmyn into the back where Michael follows and goes into Aunt Ruthies room.

"Hey, sleeping beauty, it's time to wake up. Wake up Aunt Ruthie… wake up."

"You are lucky I love you so much Michael."

"I know I am. It's time to get up."

"I'm up, I'm up. What's going on?"

"We are taking the soldiers to The Land of Dreams."

"What?"

"We are going there, because I gave them wishes for today, and they all chose everything that is there. So please get up. You must get ready, Aunt Ruthie."

"Michael, you can't take them there. They can't just up and go to a theme park. Can they?"

"Aunt Ruthie, I appreciate your concern, and you have every right to be, but today the word 'can't is not in our vocabulary. They are going to experience exactly what they want today, and what they want to be kids today."

"Are you sure?"

"Yes, Aunt Ruthie. I am. Why do you and Yolanda keep asking me that? Anyways Yolanda is getting princess ready, and so is she. So, I need you to get ready as well."

"Where is this coming from Michael?" Michael smiles.

"Again, with the questions. I need for you to trust me on this. Do you trust me?"

"Michael, if you must ask us, then you really don't understand that of course we trust you. I will get ready to leave."

"Thank you, Aunt Ruthie. I am going to get ready, and then I must pack their bags."

"Okay Michael." He then exits her room and walks down the hall.

"Hey sis!"

"Yea!"

"Can you get two extra sets of clothes and shoes for princess when you are done and put them on the table by the door for me!"

"Yes Michael!"

"Soldiers, I want you both to do the same! Did you hear me?!"

"Yes!!" Annabelle and Gabriel both shouted from their rooms as he walks into his.

"All this talk about getting ready. I should do the same. I still have the same clothes on from last night." Then he remembers the conversation he had with the angel.

"Father, how can you ask this from me? I am your servant, and I will obey all that you ask of me, but this? Father, you know in my heart that I love my children as much as I love you, even more than myself, but how can I give you one of my children? Lord, please give me the strength to follow our Father's command." He then gets showered, dressed, and ready to leave. He goes to the table by the door to gather the clothes and shoes to pack their bags.

"Okay I have their clothes and shoes. Let me just get their medicines." He goes to the kitchen cabinet.

"Okay let's see… I have their afternoon and night medicines. Just in case, I will take some extra medicine. I will grab these veggie snacks for the road." He then packs the bags and checks it over again.

"Looks like we are all packed up here. I will put these in the car so I won't forget them. Lord knows they will how excited they are." Michael puts the bags in the car, and as he walks into the house, he is greeted by everyone waiting.

"Daddy?"

"What is it buddy?"

"Where are we going?"

"Tell us Daddy! We want to know."

"It's a surprise."

"Michael, you know you can't do that to my cuties. Just tell them."

"Or I will tell my little babies."

"Okay, okay. Soldiers take a guess where we are going."

"The zoo?"

"Strike one, buddy."

"The park?"

"Strike two, sweetie."

"Just tell us. Please." The children said waiting in anticipation.

"Soldiers we are going to… The Land of Dreams!"

"Yay!!" The children shouted as Michael smiles.

"Are you all ready to have some fun?"

"Yea!" The children shouted as they exit the house.

"Okay everyone in the car." They all get in the car. "Is everyone buckled in?"

"Yea!" The children shouted.

"I am, Michael."

"Me too. Let's get on the road. I think I am more excited than the cuties." Michael smiles, and they get on the road.

"Soldiers please listen up. Can you hear me clearly back there?"

"Yea!"

"Today is your day. It will be all about you guys. I want you soldiers to go out today, have fun, and show your meanies that they won't win the fight against you all."

"Yay!!" The children shouted.

"I want you all to know that we will do whatever it is that your heart's desire, and I want you to have as much fun as possible but within your limitations. Have fun but at your own pace. Annabelle remember please don't push yourself today."

"I won't daddy."

"Me too Daddy."

"Soldiers, if for any reason you don't feel good or need a break, do not hesitate to let one of us know. Today, the theme is fun but do not be afraid to tell one of us that you are feeling ill or need to go home. We are here for you soldiers. Do not think that you are letting us down if you feel it's too much. First and foremost, we care about your health and safety. Am I clear?"

"Yes!" The children shout in excitement.

"Okay now that we got that out the way, how about we go have fun!"

"Daddy! Daddy!" The children chanted.

"Soldiers, I know that you are excited, but we will be on the road for a while. If you get hungry, let Aunt Ruthie know."

"Okay!"

"Aunt Ruthie their snacks are in their bags."

"Okay, Michael."

They make the long road trip and, after over an hour of singing and anticipation, finally arrive at the park.

"We are here soldiers!"

"Yay!!"

"Let's all get out, and I will grab the bags." Everyone exits the car.

"Soldiers, please take someone's hand."

"I with Daddy!"

"Okay buddy."

"I have Aunt Yolanda."

"And I will take my little baby Jazzy." Michael grabs their bags, and they all go to the admission window where they are greeted by a friendly employee.

"Hi! Welcome to The Land of Dreams. How many tickets do you need sir?"

"Three adults and three children please."

"What are the ages of the children sir?"

"Three, ten, and twelve."

"Okay that will be five hundred and thirty-six dollars please." Michael gives her his card through the window as she runs it. Yolanda whispers to Michael.

"Michael that is way too much. Let me pay."

"Thank you, Yolanda, but I have it handled."

"At least let me pay half."

"I appreciate that, but I invited you both here. It's my treat." Aunt Ruthie hears them talking.

"What happened?" Yolanda whispers to her. "What?! Michael we will be happy to…"

"Thank you ladies but please, I have it handled."

"Okay sir, I just need a signature."

"Okay… there you are."

"Here is your receipt and maps. Do you have any questions?"

"Just one, my children are… well let's just say they can only eat specific things." The employee realized what Michael just said.

"Oh, I am sorry to hear that, sir. Please allow me to get my manager to give you a discount on your admission."

"No, no, no. Please, I will never use my children for any gain. I was just wondering if there were any restaurants that serve protein-rich foods that are low in fat?"

"Yes, there is one that I recommend—Taste of Dreams. They bake all of their meals so there are no grease or fat in the meals, and they have sugar free deserts as well."

"Great, that sounds like winner. I was afraid there weren't any healthy options, being in a theme park and all. To be honest, this is my children's first time coming to a theme park."

"I am glad to hear you chose us for your family adventure! Although we are a theme park, and there are some other options for your choice of dining, our great chef in that particular restaurant has a very strict policy to only serve healthy alternatives for those that can't dine in our other establishments."

"Perfect, thank you so much for your help."

"My pleasure. Is there anything else I can assist you with?"

"No that's all I needed to know."

"One more thing, sir. If you need assistance for any reason, you may ask any employee here, and they will be happy to assist you. Enjoy your dreams." Michael smiles.

"Thank you so much." Michael went back to his family.

"Daddy can we go in?"

"Yeah Daddy, can we?"

"Just a second, soldiers. I need to speak with your aunts. Here, look at these maps and decide where you want to go."

"Okay!" Annabelle and Gabriel grab the maps.

"Aunt Ruthie, Yolanda, I want to start by saying how thankful that I am for both of you being here to make this happen for my soldiers. Without you two, none of this would be possible."

"You're welcome Michael."

"It's our pleasure to be with your babies."

"Today we must treat them as they are: children. You both know what they have been through for their entire lives. They have been going in and out of hospitals for God knows how long now. Today, there are no hospitals, doctors, or treatments. I want my soldiers to go out into this theme park and let their imaginations take over. I want them to experience a world other than what we had created for them at adventure land, but we must understand not to push them so hard today. I need both of you to help monitor them by watching their body language. By now both of you know how they are on good and bad days. Although they are very strong and will try to tell you that they're fine, I need both of you to step in when need be. Give them as many breaks as possible. They will try to fight you on it, and they are very smart, so just tell them you need a break or something. I already looked online at the map, and there is a medical center here that will be available if anything were to happen. Most important is their health, but other than that we must treat them as they are just children in a real theme park. Any questions?"

"I have one. What brought all this on? I ask because, although you try hard to hide it, the past three days you looked so miserable, especially yesterday. Like life was over and now suddenly this morning we pack up and come here. What's going on?"

"I agree with Yolanda, Michael. What happened between yesterday and today that would make you do this?"

"I know that I never should have to say this to you both, but please trust me in knowing this is best for my children."

"Michael, you are their father. If this is what you want, then I am with you all the way."

"As am I Michael."

"Thank you both. Now another thing to get out of the way. I know both of you are going to spoil them. Aunt Ruthie, I am looking at you."

"What? Me? No..." She said sarcastically as Michael and Yolanda laugh.

"Okay, but you both know what foods and drinks they can and can't have. If you are going to spoil them, then please do so in moderation, because they've never had junk food before, and we are in junk food city. If we separate, which more than likely we will, we will have lunch at Taste of Dreams at one. Now, if they need their medicines, you both know which ones they can have, because they are marked clearly on the labeled baggies in their bags. You must remember that in order to take their medicines, they must first eat something. Speaking of separating—Yolanda, are you okay with Annabelle?"

"Of course, I am."

"Most likely, my little buddy Gabriel will be with me, so Aunt Ruthie, that leaves you with the princess. Are you okay with that?"

"Michael, I think I can handle a three-year-old."

"Okay, but she will just want to stay in Cartoon Land. Be prepared to stay there all day with her, and please do not yell at people who stare at her neck. Most people who do not understand children's illnesses do not know how to act around them. Okay, Aunt Ruthie?"

"I got it Michael. Besides, I think I am more excited to visit Cartoon Land than Jazzy is. We will be fine."

"Okay. One more thing, Yolanda. Annabelle cannot exert herself, so please do not allow her to run around or things of that nature. No rides for anyone. Only exception is car rides like Gabriel wants to go on or any rides that are very slow. They may say that they feel okay to go on a fast ride, but it's very important that you both are my voice out here. Although they are my children, they are also yours, because we all are in this together. If at any point they feel they need their medicines, they will let you know. I know I seem like I am giving out demands or orders, but I just want this day to go so well for them. I know for a fact we will separate before lunch, and that is fine because I want them to live their dreams here. After lunch is a different story. I would very much appreciate it if we did things as a family. I want to see their beautiful smiles on their faces. I want to hear their laughter. I want to see their faces light up when we visit attractions or the animals. I want to experience what they feel. So please, and I stress this, please help me make that happen."

"Okay, Michael, we will but are you sure you are up to all this?"

"Yes Yolanda, I am. I … well, they need this day more than anything."

"Why? What is so important that they need this day?"

"Yolanda, I can't tell you why today is so important other than I need and want this day for them."

"Michael, you are kind of scaring me. What do you know that you are not telling us? Is it something one of the doctors had said?"

"No Yolanda, I need them to play and laugh as if there is no tomorrow. Okay, enough of that—let's go make memories! Hey wait! I need my camera." Yolanda laughs.

"You have a camera Michael?"

"Yes, I do."

"You know there is a camera on your phone, right?" Michael smiles.

"You know you make me feel older than I am sometimes."

"I am just saying Michael."

"I am sure my soldiers are eager to go in now."

"Yolanda, stay with the babies for a minute. I am going to speak with Michael"

"Okay." Yolanda goes to the children who are impatiently waiting.

"What do you need Aunt Ruthie?"

"You know that I love you like a son, right?"

"I do."

"Are you okay?"

"Yes, I am. I have never been happier in my life than now."

"Don't lie to me."

"I would never do that. I am telling you the truth—this is happening for my children. They can finally go to a place and roam freely and play in a world other than what they are used to."

"I don't know what you are up to Michael, but I will play along. I may be up there in years, but with that comes experience, and my experience is telling me that someone who has went through a week like you had and what your children are going through don't just up and go to a theme park."

"Aunt Ruthie, it's not just about going to play. As I keep saying over and over, this is their chance to do what most children out in the world do. Sick or not. My children are going to be just that, children. So, let's go get this started. We are wasting precious time standing here analyzing everything."

"I just want you to understand that this behavior isn't normal."

"What behavior?"

"This, Michael. What you are doing today isn't normal. When someone goes through a week like you went through, they would be calling every hospital, doctor, and clinic they can to get their children the best possible options to combat their illnesses. I'm just saying it's a concern."

"Aunt Ruthie, have faith. Yes, inside I am going through so many emotions that you wouldn't be able to imagine, but as someone just recently had told me, you must have faith. My soldiers look like they can't contain their excitement any longer. So please trust in what I am doing here. I am their father, and I promised them a genie day, so here I am granting them their wishes. So please cheer up and let's go have some fun."

"Okay Michael as long as you know what you are doing… let's go."

"Daddy! Let's go in!"

"Please Daddy!"

"Okay soldiers, let's go inside." They walk in and immediately the children are taken back.

"Wow!"

"Look at that sissy!" Michael can only smile to see the look on their faces.

"Alright soldiers, remember if you don't feel good then tell one of us."

"Okay Daddy!" The children said as they looked around.

"I know you aren't going to like this, but I want one more check."

"Daddy!" The children said in anticipation of leaving.

"Soldiers, you all know the drill."

"Fine."

"Okay."

"Head?"

"Check!"

"Tummy?"

"Check!"

"Are we done Daddy?"

"Yeah can we please do what we want?"

"Yes soldiers, you are now free to go."

"Yay!!" The children shouted with excitement.

"Princess you are with Aunt Ruthie."

"K."

"Jazzy, are you ready to go to Cartoon Land?"

"Yea!" she said, jumping up and down.

"Let's go before Daddy changes his mind."

"K."

"See you soon princess. Love you."

"Soon Daddy. Love you." she said as she and Aunt Ruthie leave.

"Annabelle, you are with Aunt Yolanda."

"Okay."

"Annabelle, where do you want to go first?"

"I want to go make a video. I want to be in one. Can we?"

"Of course, cutie. Say goodbye to your dad."

"Bye Daddy. Love you."

"I love you too sweetie."

"Let's go, cutie."

"Okay."

"Bye Michael."

"Goodbye sis." Yolanda and Annabelle begin to walk away.

"Call me if you need anything!"

"We will be fine Michael! Go race cars or something!"

"Alright buddy, looks like it's just you and me. How about we go race?"

"Yes! Imma beat you, Daddy!"

"Not if I win."

"Yeah right. You're old, Daddy." Michael laughs as they walk through the theme park.

"I bet you that I will win. What do you want to bet?" Gabriel thinks for a second.

"A pickle!"

"Out of everything here, you want a pickle?"

"Yup!" Michael laughs.

"Okay buddy, you are on."

"Alright!"

After they walked for a while, Michael finally looks at the map.

"Let's see… where are the race cars? It says we are here at Fairyland so… it should be this way. Let's go, buddy. Keep up."

"I'm here Daddy."

"How are you feeling, buddy?"

"Daddy, you don't have to keep asking me that all the time. I beat the meanies up with my magic lasers!"

"I know you did buddy, but I care about you so much."

"I know Daddy, but you don't have to worry about me because I have superpowers! Right daddy?!"

"That's right buddy, you do. You are going to show them meanies who is the boss."

"Yup!"

"Okay, the map says we should be close…"

"There it is!"

"Good job buddy. Wow, maybe you are right—I am getting old. It's a long line buddy. We may have a while before we get to race."

"Okay. I'm with you so I don't care." Michael smiles as Gabriel investigates the track, watching the cars go by.

"Daddy, look! See how fast they are going?!"

"I do buddy."

"I'm definitely going to kick your butt!"

"We shall see buddy. Just don't push yourself so hard out on the track, and please watch the other people that are racing, too."

"Okay."

"Whatever you do, don't bump me into the tires and make me crash."

"No promises." Gabriel laughs deviously.

"What was the laugh about buddy?"

"You'll see!" Michael can only do one thing and smile at his son.

"Okay buddy. Okay."

After waiting what feels like an eternity for Gabriel, it's finally their turn.

"Alright buddy, it looks like it's our turn. Are you ready?"

"Always! Imma kick your butt Daddy and get my pickle!"

"Yeah, yeah, talk is cheap buddy. Show me on the track."

"Oh, I will!"

They walk onto the track and are greeted by one of the racetrack crew.

"Hey guys, are you ready to race?"

"Yup! Imma beat my daddy!" The employee laughs.

"Yeah it looks like you are ready."

"Oh, I am!"

Michael pulls the crew member close. "Excuse me sir?"

"What can I help you with?"

"How safe are these karts? And how fast do they run? I am asking for my son. You know how we parents are."

"That's perfectly fine, sir. Don't worry, the kart that we will put him in is a special kart for children his age. They don't run fast, and we test the karts before opening and after closing every day. We also inspect the track, safety latches, and helmets after every race. We do all this to ensure our guests have a safe, good time here. Your son will have a safe race with you and apparently beat you." Michael and the employee laughs.

"Yeah he wants to win."

"I will get your son into his kart."

"Thank you."

"Okay little guy I have a special kart just for you right here."

"Alright! Look Daddy! It's red like your favorite team!"

"Hey that's not fair. I want that one!"

"No! It's mine!" The employee helps Gabriel get into his kart and put on his helmet as another employee helps Michael to his.

"Hi, how are you doing, sir?"

"I am good, and you?"

"I love the smell of the track, so I am living the dream here."

"Well that's good. At least you get to do what you love."

"This kart is for you, sir."

"Thank you. Wait, I need to go strap my son in."

"That's okay we take care of all that sir. My fellow pit crew member is helping him to make sure he is in there nice and tight and that your son will have a safe race."

"I'm sorry it's just I am like any parent, and I worry about my children. He hasn't been feeling well and today is a great day for him and that is why we are here."

"That's understandable, sir. We have a kill switch that someone maintains every race. We also are out here monitoring the races, so if we notice anything wrong, we will shut off his kart with no problem. We also have standby medical professional in the off-chance that someone needs medical attention."

"That's very assuring to hear. Wow, you all do not play around when it comes to safety here."

"No sir, we do not. We care about the safety and well-being of all of our guests."

"I must send your office a nice thank-you card for doing such a terrific job here. Now I am truly sorry that I tried to butt in on your procedures."

"That's quite alright sir, and we really do appreciate your feedback. Okay, looks like your son is strapped in and so are you. We will check the other drivers, and at the green light you may race."

"Thank you, sir."

"It's our pleasure. Enjoy the race."

"Thank you. Hey buddy, are you ready?!"

"Yup! Are you ready to get me my pickle?!" Michael laughs.

"Yes, son I am ready!"

"Good!"

"Hey buddy!"

"Yeah!"

"Wait for the green light!"

"Okay! I'm ready already!" Gabriel turns to look at Michael.

"Buddy, pay attention!"

"Okay!"

"Look it's on red, yellow, and…"

"Green! Woohoo!" Michael tried to keep his eyes on the track but couldn't help looking at the joy on his son's face as he went around the track.

"Daddy! Look at me! Look how fast I'm going!"

"Go buddy! Go!"

"Woohoo!!"

After many laps around the track and once where Michael of course crashed, the race ends, and they both exit their karts. He sees the excitement in his son's face.

"Daddy did you see me?!"

"I did buddy."

"I was going *vroom*! I was going so fast!"

"I know buddy, you were going so fast that you beat me." Gabriel laughs.

"I told you I was going to kick your butt Daddy!"

"That you did buddy. I had you in the second-to-last turn, then the tires came out of nowhere and hit my kart!"

"Ha-ha you crashed Daddy! I told you, you were old!"

"Listen here buddy I have your old right here!" Michael tickles Gabriel as he giggles.

"I will give it to you buddy, you beat me."

"Yeah I did!"

"Are you ready to collect your winnings?"

"Yup! Pickle time!" They exit the track.

"You know I must ask buddy…"

"Yeah Daddy, my tummy is good."

"Sorry buddy, but you know how I am."

"I know. Can we go get my pickle now?!"

"Yes, buddy we can."

"Yes!"

"Tell me buddy, what is it with this pickle? You have a free ticket to get any junk food here, and you want this pickle?"

"I heard some people that visited my friend at Adventure Land, and he told him about all these pickles here, and I really want to try one."

"Really?"

"Yup! And guess what?"

"What?"

"They even have juices in them."

"Buddy all pickles have juice in them."

"Not these ones. These have juices like the ones you dink at the store!"

"Is that true buddy?"

"Yup!"

"Okay buddy let's go get you one."

"Yes!"

After searching throughout the park, Michael finally goes up to an employee.

"Excuse me miss?"

"Hi, what can I help you with?"

"My son here heard of these apparently amazing pickles. Can you direct us where we may find these magic pickles?" The employee smiles.

"Yes sir, they are just right over there by the gift store. It's called Ava's Pickle Land; you can find them in there." As the employee points behind Michael, he notices how close they were and is embarrassed.

"Oh okay. Maybe I should take the time to look around before I ask." He and the employee laugh.

"It's quite alright sir. Enjoy your time here at The Land of Dreams, and if you have any more questions, we are always delighted to answer them."

"Thank you so much. You have a great day."

"Thank you, sir. Bye little guy."

"Bye." Gabriel waves as they walk toward the store.

"You heard her buddy, let's go in here to get your winnings."

"Yes!"

Michael opens the door for his son. "After you buddy. You are the winner."

"Thank you."

"You're welcome buddy."

They enter the store and are greeted by a friendly employee.

"Hi there, welcome to Ava's Pickle Land. Is there something I can help you find?"

"Yes hi, my little buddy here for some reason is hypnotized on getting a pickle from here."

"Well, we do have the best pickles in Florida. We have all kinds and flavors."

"Flavors? My son told me about juices. I believe everything my son tells me, but to be honest, I was a little skeptical, because he had heard it from a friend. I thought it was just a pickle that someone had spilled their juice in."

"No, actually we had launched a wide variety garlic, hot, juice flavored. Basically, you can make pickles with whatever flavor you can think of."

"Wow, that's amazing."

"Daddy look! They have fruit punch!"

"Not fruit punch buddy!" Michael said jokingly.

"Yup!"

"Well, I guess he knows exactly what he wants."

"Excellent choice! That's our most popular with big guys like you!" Gabriel bashfully giggles.

"Okay we will take I guess fruit punch then."

"Excellent, and for you sir?"

"Oh no I am okay. Thank you."

"Daddy, you have to get one!"

"Yes sir. If you say so. I guess make that two of them."

"Great choice. Don't worry, you will enjoy it. Do you need a bag?"

"That's not necessary. I am sure his will be gone before we make it 10 feet from the store." They both laugh.

"Okay sir, that will be $21.50."

"Here is my card… It's chipped, so do I just insert it in the little machine here?"

"Yes sir."

"Sorry, technology and I don't mix well."

"It happens to us all."

"Yeah tell me about it. I hear it all the time." The employee smiles.

"Here is your receipt sir. Thank you for stopping by today. Have a wonderful day."

"Thank you. May you have a blessed day."

"Bye big guy."

"Bye. Thank you." Gabriel waved as they exited the store and headed to a bench.

"Alright buddy, let's have a seat here and enjoy our pickles."

"Okay."

"Need help opening your…" He sees Gabriel enjoying his pickle.

"Oh, I guess that answers that."

"Mm." Michael smiles.

"Well I might need help opening mine buddy."

"Just rip it Daddy."

"Okay buddy, I got it. Do I even have to ask how is it?"

"Nope!"

"Okay buddy, may I ask you something?"

"Sure."

"What do you want in life?"

"Huh?"

"For example, what do you want to be when you grow up?"

"Like you Daddy!"

Michael's heart fills with love and smiles.

"I love you, son."

"I love you too, Daddy, but why do you keep calling me your son? I'm your little buddy!"

"Yes, you are my little buddy but the type of person that I am, as your father, I want you to always remember that you are someone's son. Never forget that. Okay?"

"Okay."

"Going back to the subject, what do you want to have in life?"

"I want the meanies to go away. I want to ride cars and have a little buddy like me!"

"That sounds good to me."

"Daddy?"

"Yes buddy?"

"Will the meanies ever go away from my tummy?" Gabriel asked with his head down, and Michael instantly remembered what he and the angel had discussed.

"Yes, buddy they will. I promise that soon that all of you will be cured from the meanies. None of you will ever feel any pain from the meanies. No more doctors or magic potions and lasers."

"Promise Daddy?"

"Do you trust me?"

"Yeah."

"Then believe me when I say this: Everything that you soldiers are going through will vanish. Just like that!" Michael snapped his fingers, and Gabriel looks on with excitement.

"Really Daddy?!"

"I promise buddy, but I need you to understand something. Sometimes in order to see that beautiful rainbow in the sky that you love so much it must first what?"

"Rain?"

"Exactly buddy. Do you understand what I am saying to you?"

"Yeah, but what if it rains forever?"

"It won't buddy."

"How do you know?"

"Because it was promised to us from our Father, and a sign of that promise is a rainbow after it rains."

"That's awesome!"

"It is buddy. I will also promise to you as your father. Yes, it may rain in your life, and it will seem like you are caught in the middle of a storm, and all you see is darkness everywhere, but in the end there will be no need for umbrellas, no more dark days in your life. When it is all over with, the son will appear and shine ever so brightly in your life, and at that moment you will be able to look up in the sky and see that beautiful rainbow of yours."

"Really?!"

"I promise buddy."

"Thanks Daddy."

"You are welcome, buddy. It's time for me to call your aunts and check in with them."

"Okay."

Michael takes out his phone and calls Yolanda first.

"Hello?"

"Hey sis. I was just checking in. How is it going on your end?"

"Michael, you should see your daughter, the movie star!"

"What?"

"Yeah, you know how they let them make videos and stuff? Well, she is the star of the show! It's so cute."

"Really? I can't believe I am missing out on that."

"Michael, trust me she isn't going anywhere. We will be here for a while."

"Okay, my buddy and I are going to make a couple of stops, then we will head right over there."

"By the time you do that, won't it be time for lunch?"

"Wow you are right about that. See I knew you were for here for a reason." Michael laughs.

"How is she doing with her…"

"She is fine Michael. You were right. I have never seen her light up like this before. I will send you a video of her."

"See this is what I was talking about. I didn't want to miss out on that kind of excitement."

"We have all day, Michael. I am sure she will be more than happy to show off her movie talent to you."

"Okay sis, I will see you all soon at lunch."

"Okay Michael, we will meet me you guys at one."

"Okay sis I will see you both at the restaurant."

"Bye, Michael."

"What is sissy doing, Daddy?"

"Apparently, she is becoming a movie star."

"Cool!"

"Let's see how Aunt Ruthie is doing with Jazzy."

"Okay."

He then calls her.

"Hello?"

"Hey, Aunt Ruthie. I am just checking in and seeing how you and princess are doing."

"Were having a good time over here. She can't get enough of these cartoon characters."

"Wow it does sound like she is having a good time."

"Trust me she is."

"That's good to hear. How is she doing health wise?"

"She is good Michael. I have been watching her closely."

"Great, well there is nothing more to say other than I will see you both at the restaurant at one for lunch."

"Sounds good to me. I can't wait. That's if I can drag her away from this place."

"Please find some way because I want to be there."

"Michael I was joking."

"Oh, I apologize."

"It's okay Michael. Well see you all in a bit."

"Okay Aunt Ruthie, I will see both of you at one."

"Bye Michael." He hangs up the phone.

"What's Jazzy doing, Daddy?"

"She is having fun over at Cartoon Land."

"I love genie day Daddy!"

"I am glad you do and that your sisters are having fun as well."

"What are we doing next Daddy?"

"We are here for you, so you tell me."

"I want to play video games and shoot some bad guys!"

"Okay buddy, your wish is my command. The arcade center is just over here."

They walk into the arcade.

"Okay buddy, are you ready?"

"Yup!"

"Let's go shoot some bad guys."

"Yes!"

After they play many games, Michael realizes that it's time for them to leave.

"Buddy, I know that you are having fun, but we must leave so that we can go have lunch."

"Okay."

They exit and head for the restaurant.

"Wow that was a lot of games huh buddy?"

"Yeah it was!"

"Which one was your favorite?"

"Watching you trying to run from the monsters. That was funny."

"Hey, those monsters were coming out of nowhere."

"I liked the motorcycle game, too."

"You did look pretty good up there. You looked like you knew what you were doing."

"I want one!"

"Slow down buddy, you must crawl before you walk."

"Huh?"

Michael smiles. "Nothing buddy. We better hurry and meet everyone. We were in that arcade longer than I thought."

"I want to play more games. Can we Daddy?"

"Buddy I know today is your day, but you need some fuel in you."

"But I can eat another pickle."

"I'm afraid not buddy. I want everyone to eat together as a family. That's very important to me."

"Why Daddy?"

"Gabriel, always remember that no matter how much is going on in your life, always make time for your family. You understand what I am saying?"

"Yeah, yeah."

"Buddy…"

"I understand."

"It's okay, buddy. I know that you might not understand me clearly now because you are having so much fun, but one day you will."

They then walk up to the restaurant, and Michael notices his aunt.

"Look buddy, it's Aunt Ruthie and your sister."

"Daddy!!" Jazmyn said running to him.

"Hi Princess."

"Hi."

"Are you having fun?"

"Yeah."

"What about you, Aunt Ruthie?"

"I am having a great time here."

"That's good. Is she keeping you busy?"

"She is having such a good time here that she wouldn't be able to pick me out of a line up."

"Awesome. I wonder where Annabelle and Yolanda could be?"

"Probably lost track of time. You know how this place is."

"I know, but I wanted for all of us to eat together as a family."

"Here they come, Michael."

Yolanda and Annabelle walk up.

"Hey ladies, are we having fun?"

"Lots of fun, Daddy!"

"I am glad you are, sweetie."

"Oh my gosh Michael, you have to see this video of your daughter…" Yolanda pulls up the video. "Look how natural she is."

"Wow sweetie you look like you are made to be in movies."

"Daddy!" Annabelle said, embarrassed.

"I'm serious sweetie. One day you are going to be up there on the big screen, and we all are going to pay just to see your movies."

"That's my dream Daddy."

"Never lose that dream sweetie. Soldiers, are you ready for lunch?"

"Yeah!" The children shouted.

"Okay, I know I am hungry. What about you two ladies?"

"I'm starving."

"So am I."

"Everyone, please listen up. This place is a buffet style restaurant."

"What's that Daddy?"

"Buddy, it means that you get to pick out whatever you are hungry for. They pretty much have anything that your big heart desires."

"Awesome!"

"It is buddy. When we walk in here do not be afraid to get what you want, and I want everyone to be good and full, because after you are full it will be time for your medicines. So, eat up."

"Okay!" The children shouted as the family walked into the restaurant.

"Oh wow, it's so beautiful in here."

"I love the paintings on the walls."

"I should hope so ladies. After all, it is called Taste of Dreams."

"You're right about the paintings, Aunt Ruthie. I love how the murals all blend with the theme here. It doesn't stick out but at the same it's not buried."

The children look on in amazement at the food.

"Wow, look at all the food! Daddy look! They have spaghetti!"

"Look Daddy! Pizza!"

Michael smiles.

"I knew your eyes would have spotted those. Go ahead and grab as much as you would like. If you want more, than feel free to come back and get another plate. I want you all to be good and full."

"Okay!" The children happily grabbed plates.

"Princess look, they have chicken nuggets and French fries. Would you like that?"

"Mm." Michael laughs.

"Well that answers that."

"Michael how does this work?"

"Well sis, we pick our selection, and when we are finished, we pay up front at the cashier before we may sit."

"Oh, I thought it was like a buffet."

"No, I just said that to explain to them that you can pick whatever you want. So, if you do want more you can just come back up here and repeat the process."

"Oh, okay."

"Hey Michael, are you sure these babies can handle all this type of food?"

"It's perfectly fine, Aunt Ruthie. We are in the Taste of Dreams, remember? We of course must watch their intake but today's free game."

"Okay Michael, but I am not helping you clean out the car when they get sick." She smiled and so did Michael.

"That is why God invented vacuums."

"I want you to do whatever it is that you are doing for your children, but you must remember that they are sick, Michael."

"I appreciate your concern, Aunt Ruthie, but look at them over there, without a care in the world. Besides, I will let you in on a secret. This restaurant has strict policies on what they serve. The chefs bake all the meals. So, everything you see here has no fat or grease. They ensure that guests like my soldiers that can't eat at other establishments here at the park have healthy alternatives. But shh, don't tell them that."

"Well, I was a little concerned that you threw your cautions out the window by coming here, but I'm very proud of you on how you are giving them this experience but at the same time keeping in mind that they have these illnesses. That's very admirable." They both smiled.

"Well thank you, Aunt Ruthie. That means a lot."

After everyone gets their meals and drinks, Michael gathers everyone.

"Okay soldiers, ladies, we must pay the toll before we may sit."

They walk up to a friendly cashier.

"Hi folks, how many in your party?"

"Hi, there are three adults and three children. Do we need to weigh our plates or something?"

"No sir, we just charge by the plate. The drinks are included."

"Oh, I apologize, I thought it was by weight."

"That's understandable sir, most guests think that as well. Don't worry, you are not the only one, it happens more often than you think."

"That's makes me feel better." He and the cashier laugh.

"What's the damage?"

"Your total is $76.96."

"Before my brother tries to pay and argue with me, please take my card."

As the cashier smiles, she takes her card.

"Sis what are you doing?"

"Hush Michael. Just go get us a table."

"Thank you, sis. Okay soldiers let's go find us a table."

The children hold their plates and follow Michael as he chooses a table.

"Okay soldiers, this looks like a good spot. Please have a seat."

As they all sat down, Michael realized that Jazmyn wasn't big enough to sit at the table.

"Oh, I'm sorry princess. I will grab you a special chair just for you. Aunt Ruthie do you mind…"

"Go Michael."

"Thank you."

He goes up to an employee.

"Excuse me?"

"Hi, what can I help you with today sir?"

"Yes, I was wondering if there were any highchairs available?"

"Absolutely sir. Which table are you dining at?" Michael points to his table where Yolanda has put down her plate and drink. "Right over there where my sister just sat down."

"I will be right over with one, sir."

"It's okay I can just take it."

"You are our guest, sir. I will be more than happy to bring it for you."

"I appreciate that." Michael walks over, and as he sits the employee brings the highchair.

"Here you are, sir. Is there anything else that you and your family will be needing, sir?"

"I think that will be it. I thank you so much for that."

"My pleasure sir. You all enjoy your meals."

"Thank you. Okay princess, let's get you in your chair." Michael picks her up. "Let me just get you in here, fasten these straps, and... there you are princess, you are all set to eat."

"Mm..."

"I can't wait to eat my pizza!"

"Yeah, my spaghetti looks yummy!"

"I know that you all can't wait to eat, but you know what we must do first."

"But Daddy, everyone can see us."

"Sweetie, never feel ashamed of loving God, because he is never ashamed of loving you. We must always thank him for everything that he blesses us with. Are we not thankful that we are here? That we can eat together as a family at this restaurant?"

"Yes, but nobody else is." Michael smiles.

"Then sweetie why not be the first?"

"You're right, Daddy. I'm sorry."

"That's okay sweetie. I tell you what, how about we all give thanks in our own way."

"Okay but in our heads?"

"Sweetie, I cannot make you give thanks. That is something you must do on your own. So, if that is your way of giving thanks, then by all means do so. If you thank our Father in your heart, that is all he asks of you."

"Okay Daddy I can do that."

"Me too, Daddy."

"Great, so when you all are finished you may eat."

The children bowed their heads as does everyone else at the table. Michael closes his eyes and says grace.

"Heavenly Father, we are very thankful for today and this meal that you have blessed us with. I am especially thankful that you allowed this day to happen. In your heavenly name Jesus, I pray. Amen." Michael opens his eyes and notices everyone staring at him.

"Okay everyone, what are we waiting for? Let's eat!"

"Pizza!"

"Mm."

Michael laughs as he sits and watches his children. "Wow Aunt Ruthie, hungry, are we?" he said jokingly.

"Hey, you run around with a three-year-old and see if you don't work up an appetite." Everyone laughs.

"I hear you. So, soldiers, what's next on the schedule for you guys?"

"I want to race again!"

"I want to see the animals!"

"Sounds ambitious, but I hate that we are not spending this day as a family. I have an idea. After we all finish with our meals, we spend the rest of the day together. All of us. So that we may experience everything this park has to offer."

"But Daddy, I want to go with Aunt Yolanda again and go see the..." Yolanda looks into Michael's eyes and sees that what she just said hurt him.

"Hey cutie, how about you show your brother and sister how to star in a video, and all three of you cuties can be in one together, and then Gabriel, you can race your sister. How does that sound?"

"Oh, sissy I'm going to beat you like I did Daddy!"

"I bet you won't!"

Michael can only do one thing as he looks over to his sister. "Thank you, Yolanda. I really appreciate that."

"Family. Right Michael?"

"Yes sis, family. What about you princess?"

"Oh, she doesn't care where we go, Michael. She is just happy to be here."

"Okay, it's settled. After we finish, we will enjoy this park together, as a family."

Some time goes by, and they all finish their meals. Michael then gathers all the plates and an employee comes and picks them up.

"I will take these plates and cups if you are all finished."

"Yes, we are finished with the plates, but we need the cups still."

"I will be happy to take the plates and when you are finished with your glasses, you may leave them on the table, and I will come and collect them"

"It's okay I can dispose of them. Where do I set them?"

"You are very special guests of ours. We will be delighted to."

"You all have such great hospitality here. I thank you for that."

"My pleasure. Enjoy the rest of your day."

"Thank you. Okay soldiers, are we good and full?"

"That was good pizza!"

"I'm glad you enjoyed it, sweetie."

"My tummy hurts a little, Daddy."

"I was waiting for that buddy. It's time for your medicines. It looks like you all have drinks left so…" Michael pulls out their medicines. "Here is something to help you soldiers. Here you go buddy."

"Thank you, Daddy."

"You're welcome, and sweetie here are yours…"

"Thank you."

"You're welcome. Aunt Ruthie, do you mind giving princess hers?"

"Sure. Here you go baby."

"All gone."

"Mine too, Daddy."

"Very good soldiers."

"Gone."

"Good job princess. We are going to sit for a minute and let your medicines beat up the meanies."

"Hey Michael, let's, you, me, and Aunt Ruthie talk over here for a second."

"Sure sis. Soldiers, we are just going to be over here, so look at your maps and see where you would like to go."

"Okay!" The children look at the maps.

"What's going on ladies?"

"Michael, no one will judge you if we cut it short today and head home. They had fun. We all did."

"I cannot stress this enough that they need this."

"Or is it that you need this Michael? Aunt Ruthie and I are with you 100 percent, but it's okay if we head home now."

"If I felt that we needed to head home, we would. I will never put my children's health in jeopardy just for a theme park, but look how happy they are over there. They need this day more than anything to be children. To laugh and play like they are."

"Michael, son, we have tomorrow, if you are up for it, we can come back. Let them go home and recover."

"That's the problem. Aunt Ruthie, Yolanda, the way everything's headed, I'm afraid tomorrow is not an option."

"Michael don't ever talk like that!"

"I'm sorry Yolanda. I have so much on my mind that I cannot think straight. I really need you both to put your trust in me."

"Michael, we can help you. As always, Yolanda and I are here for you and those babies of yours. We can help, only if you will just inform us of what is going on. Talk to us Michael."

"From the bottom of my heart I thank you both for always being around when we need you, but I'm afraid somethings are better left unsaid. I will say this—I have a strong feeling that my family will be going through a storm soon, and I need both of you for guiding this family through it. I need your words that no matter what may come that you both will never lose your faiths."

"Of course, Michael."

"Anything you and those cuties need."

"Thank you both. So, how about we take on this park some more. I'm sure my soldiers can't wait." They go back to the table.

"How are feeling soldier?"

"Good!"

"I feel better too, Daddy!"

"Great! Are you soldiers ready to have more fun?"

"Yeah!!" the children shout with excitement.

"Okay let's get to it."

They walked the park for hours admiring all the exhibits, visiting one attraction to another. Michael couldn't help but admire the laughter in his children's voices. The way their faces lit up seeing all the wonders around them. The life they have in their eyes. His heart fills with so many emotions that he could only turn to his sister and speak softly.

"Look at them, Yolanda. Forget yesterday, forget tomorrow. Today is what I want them to remember. Being here with those that love them dearly. Having these memories that will last a lifetime is all I ever wanted them to have."

"You were right, and they do have these memories, and they have us to never let them forget it."

"Yolanda, Aunt Ruthie, I need you to promise me that you will never forget."

"I promise Michael."

"I give you my word Michael."

"There aren't enough words to describe how thankful I am that both of you helped this happen."

"It was our pleasure, Michael."

Michael smiles as they reach the end of the park and wait for the fireworks show to end the night.

"Okay soldiers, the fireworks are about to start. Do you all have a good view?"

"Where are they Daddy?"

"I can't see them?"

"Just look up soldiers, and you will see the magic of this theme park turning the dark sky into light. Just believe in it and you will see it."

"Okay!" the children said as they investigated the sky in anticipation.

"Where Daddy?"

"Trust me buddy, it's there. Just wait. You will see it."

At that moment, silence fell upon everyone there in attendance viewing. Then, out of nowhere, the once dark sky lit up and they heard the first sound. Boom!

"Wow Daddy! I see it! Look!"

"I see it too, buddy"."

"I see it Daddy!"

"I know you do, sweetie."

Michael couldn't take his eyes of his children as all three stood there point-
ing, laughing, and looking on in amazement at the sky as one by one crack-
les and pops hit the night sky. In that moment, he knew that soon one
will see something far more wonderful. One will be singing, dancing with
angles. One will be walking with Jesus. One will be with our Father in the
kingdom of heaven. As he looked up into the heavens to watch, the last of
the fireworks had been released and just as it was light, the sky returned to
darkness again. The night had ended. As they began to make their way to
the car his children were still fired up from what they just saw.

"Daddy did you see that?!"

"I did see something wonderful buddy."

"It went *boom*! And *pow!*" Michael just smiles.

"I was there too buddy."

"It was awesome!"

"Daddy that was amazing!"

"I am glad you liked it sweetie."

"But it was dark, then suddenly, everything looked like it was daylight!
How did they do that?!"

"Magic, sweetie."

"Daddy… I'm serious."

"Well, I tell you what, listen up soldiers. It's just like in life. At first everything will seem dark and quiet then, out of nowhere, your life will be lit up
for you to see your way through. You must always have faith and believe
in our Father, in yourselves, and in each other. With that your lives will be
lit forever."

"Awesome!"

"Like right now, Daddy, we are sick but then everything will get better?!"

"Exactly right sweetie. Nothing stays dark forever. For if you put your trust in God and allow Him to be your light, soldiers, you will always see."

"Okay Daddy!" the children said as they make it to the car.

"Wow it's late. It's time for you all to take your medicines before we make the long trip home. I'm sure glad I bought these drinks on the way out. Here you are soldiers."

As they each they take their medicines, they are still pumped up for the day and can only shout out a sentence before they get into the car.

"Yay! Best day ever!!"

As the children get in the car, Yolanda and Aunt Ruthie turn to Michael.

"Today was a good day, Michael. Thank you for letting us experience this day with your cuties."

"You're welcome sis."

"Michael, I wouldn't have missed this day for the world. Thank you."

Michael smiles at them. "You're welcome, Aunt Ruthie, and thank you both for today. Let's get on this long road trip home. I need to get them in bed."

"I am certain that they will fall asleep before we even get on the road, Michael."

"Them?! I think I will be the first one out!"

As they all share a laugh Michael responds.

"Aunt Ruthie, don't go off and show your age now."

"Hey, it's way past my bedtime, but I wouldn't change a thing. I am glad we came."

"I agree."

"Okay ladies, let's head home."

They get into the car, and as they begin to leave, Michael notices how quickly his children went from excited to exhausted.

"Hey soldiers are you okay back there?"

"I'm tired Daddy."

"Me too."

"Okay soldiers, rest up while we go home."

"Okay…" they said, closing their eyes.

They then get on the main road for the long journey home. Yolanda looks at everyone, then turns to Michael and softly speaks.

"Well that didn't take long. Even Aunt Ruthie is sleeping."

"Yeah… they had a big day."

"We all did, but it was fun."

"I know it was a great day, sis. Thanks again for today."

"Anytime Michael. Maybe next time they can actually ride the rides."

At that moment, it hit Michael that he knew in fact that his children will be healthy enough to do so but must first endure the pain that will soon come.

"Michael, don't look so worried. Everything will be okay. Just as today's memories happened, many more will come. Just continue to pray and stay with your faith."

"I know, Yolanda, and that's not the issue. I have faith, and as I tell my soldiers all the time to believe and have faith, I do personally know that everything will in fact be okay."

"Then that is all that needs to be said, Michael. With that in mind you will see brighter days. I am going to rest my eyes now. I can't wait to get home."

"Okay, sis."

Michael has that word in his mind—home—and whispers, "But who will it be?"

"Did you say something Michael?"

"No, sis, rest up. I am just thinking out loud."

"Okay, wake me when we get there."

"Okay, sis."

As time passes by and as Michael drives farther down the road, silence goes throughout the car, and his mind replays the conversation he had with the angel. As he does that, thoughts he never wanted to come into his mind started pouring in. Every hug, smile, every "daddy" that his children did or said starts to get to him, and he starts to talk to our Father in his mind.

"Father, why must you task me with such a decision? It's not fair that come midnight on Sunday, I must give you my decision on which of my children will return home with you. Which is the one who I will not see grow? Which is the one that will be without their family here on Earth? I understand that you want us all to return home Father, but why now? Why do you want one of my children? Forgive me Father, for I am no one to question you. I am your servant, and if this is thy will, then with all my strength, I will obey. As much as it will weaken me, and I know it will weaken my family as well, Father, I know you will be there guiding my family through this pain. I know this is more like a complaint than a prayer I must say in your heavenly name Jesus I pray, Amen."

Just like that, they arrive home. Michael sits there in his car and looks at everyone sleeping, and he knew in his heart that this day may in fact had been the last thing they all did together. As a family. He then speaks softly to his sister and aunt.

"Hey sis... Aunt Ruthie... Were home. We must get them inside"

"Okay, Michael. I will grab Annabelle. Aunt Ruthie you get Jazzy."

They all get inside, and one by one Michael puts his children in their beds, hugging them ever so tightly, then kisses each one as he lays them in their beds. He then stands at the end of the hallway looking on to each of them in their rooms. He can only think of one thing to say.

"I love you all so much in a way that I can't even express it. Goodnight my soldiers."

He goes out to the living room where his sister and aunt are.

"Are their bags in the house?"

"Yeah, we grabbed them and locked the car doors and yes before you ask, I had already locked the house door and set the alarm."

"Thank you, sis."

"Michael, I have a bed that is calling my name. Goodnight you two."

"Goodnight, Aunt Ruthie. I love you."

"Goodnight, Aunt Ruthie. I love you, too."

"I love you both as well. Goodnight." She then goes into her room.

"Wow what a day. I am beat. I am going to bed now."

"Okay, sis. Goodnight."

"You're not going to bed Michael?"

"No sis, I am just going to sit in my chair and think for a while."

"Okay Michael but get some rest."

"Okay, sis. Love you."

"I love you too, Michael. Goodnight." She goes into her room.

Michael sits in the very chair that he had the conversation with the angel and once again his mind starts to race, only this time it's about his children's illnesses. He starts to wonder which of his children benefits from this decision. Which of his children has a better chance at life? He then answers his own questions—they all do. They all will benefit from this, but if one must return home then.…

His phone rings and he answers, puzzled.

"Hello?"

"Hi Michael, it's Jessica"

"Oh, hi."

"Is this a bad time? I know I am calling you pretty late at night."

"No, you're fine, you just caught me off guard. How are you?"

"I'm good, but from the sound of your voice I should be asking you that."

"Sorry about that. We had a busy day today. We took my soldiers to a theme park today and came home not too long ago. I'm just sitting here thinking about something things."

"At Adventure Land?"

"No, we went to a real theme park."

"That's good. Which one?"

"Land of Dreams."

"That's a good choice. Did you guys have fun today?"

"It was a great day. You should have seen my soldiers. They laughed, played. They were able to be children today. They had a blast."

"I'm glad to hear that. I'm also glad they have a father like you that can give them that."

"I wouldn't say that, but yes today was a blessing. I just have so much on my mind now."

"What's on your mind?"

"I know I opened the door by saying that but only if I could tell you Jessica."

"Well try to. What's going on?"

"It's just … well… never mind it's nothing."

"You can't start to say something, Michael, and then say it's nothing. Just tell me what you wanted to say."

"Well, have you ever been given a blessing, then when you analyze it, it feels more like a curse?"

"Many of times, but how do you feel you have a more of a curse than blessing?"

"The blessing is that I have an opportunity to heal my children, but the curse is it comes with a high price tag."

"Great! Then do it, Michael. What is there to think about?"

"It's not that simple Jessica."

"Do what I do when I am faced with that type of feeling. Pray on it."

"Believe me, I have prayed on it, and I am afraid that is what led me to this point."

"Michael, all you can do is to pray, have faith, and then you will know that no matter what comes from it, it was our Father who led you to that point."

"That's what I am afraid of."

"Listen Michael, whatever it is that you must do to heal your children, then trust in our Father to guide you. With that you will never be lost."

"Thank you for that it's just…" Michael hears a loud scream coming from one of his children's rooms.

Chapter 11

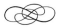

"Daddy!!"

Michael hears the cry again.

"Daddy!!"

Michael drops the phone and immediately rushes to the cry. He scrambles to the cry to find it's coming from Gabriel's room, and as he rushes inside his room, he finds Gabriel clutching his stomach.

"Gabriel! What's wrong?!"

"I don't know, it hurts! I'm scared Daddy!"

"Don't worry Gabriel, Daddy's here. Let me get the doctor on the phone."

Michael, panicky, searches for his phone.

"Where is my phone?!"

"Daddy please it hurts!" he cries in anguish as Michael tries to calm him down.

"It's going to be okay buddy. I will take you to the hospital."

"Daddy it hurts!" He continues to cry and Michael shouts for Yolanda.

"Yolanda! Yolanda!" She comes rushing in and notices Gabriel crying.

"What's going on?"

"I don't know, he is in a lot of pain. I am taking him to the hospital to get checked out."

"Okay I will stay with the girls."

"Thank you."

At that moment, Michael hears another scream.

"Daddy!!"

"Yolanda, stay with Gabriel."

"Okay."

"Daddy, hurry!"

"Annabelle I'm coming!"

Michael rushes to her room to find her vomiting, clutching her chest.

"Annabelle!"

"Daddy, make it stop! Tell them to stop squeezing my chest!" she cries out.

"What?! Annabelle tell me what is going on?!"

"It hurts so…" She faints.

"Annabelle! Annabelle talk to me!" Michael screams to her as she lay there, then he shouts to his sister.

"Yolanda! Call nine one-one!"

"I already did! They are on their way!"

His aunt rushes into Annabelle's room.

"Michael what's going on?" As she sees Michael crying, clutching Annabelle, she is in shock.

"Oh, my lord. What happened?!"

"I don't know. First Gabriel is in a great deal of pain, then Annabelle calls out for me and now… she is just laying here! I don't know what is happening!" Michael cries out. "Oh God, please not now!"

"I will get Jazmyn!"

"Please go check on her. Please!"

"Okay Michael, okay." She rushes into Jazmyn's room. "Hey Jazzy… Jazmyn wake up." As she nudges Jazmyn, she notices she is not waking up. "Jazmyn?… Jazmyn! Michael, she is not getting up!"

What?!" Michael franticly screams out. "Somebody tell me what is happening?!" He then hears sirens outside his house and pounding on the door.

"I will get the door!" Yolanda shouts as she rushes to the door.

"Hurry!" Michael's once quiet house is now filled with emergency personnel. He hears a voice.

"Sir. Sir."

"Help her! Help my children!"

"Calm down, sir, we are here to help. What happened?"

"I don't know! My son cried out to me, and when I went to him, he was clutching his chest saying he is in pain. Then my daughter cried out to me, and as I came in, she was vomiting, saying that her chest felt like someone was squeezing it, then just collapsed! My aunt went to check on my youngest and now she isn't waking up! What are you guys doing?! Please do something!" As he described to them what has happened the other personnel go into his children's rooms. They begin to examine Annabelle.

"Sir, we will tend to your children, and we called for additional units, but you must remain calm."

"Calm?! Calm! How can you say that?! Help my children! Please!"

"Sir we are. What did she say or do before she collapsed?"

"She was clutching her chest, vomiting, then just collapsed!"

"Do your children suffer from any illnesses or allergies?"

"Yes, she has progeria, my son has DSRCT, and my youngest has neuroblastoma. They all go for treatments at Tampa Cancer Center. They have their own doctors there. Help them please!"

"Sir, we are doing everything we can, but I need you to give us some space so that we may see what is happening."

Michael franticly runs from room to room and then stands in the hallway and shouts out to heaven.

"God! Please help my children!"

"Sir we are working on them, please allow us to do so."

"What?!"

Yolanda and Aunt Ruthie see Michael panicking and crying. They go to him to calm him down.

"Michael, let them handle this. They are trained professionals. They know what they are doing."

"Yolanda, this is all my fault!" Michael, feeling the guilt, cries and speaks softly. "I shouldn't had pushed them so hard today. Only if we had stayed home… then none of this would be happening."

His aunt speaks. "Michael, regardless if it was because we went there or not, with their illnesses these things may happen no matter what they do."

"I'm so sorry…"

Michael is taken from all the emotions he is feeling and drops to his knees.

"Michael, I know that this is overwhelming, but you must get it together. They are very strong children. They aren't gone, Michael. They are still here."

"At least for now, Aunt Ruthie, they are."

"What?!" Yolanda says in disbelief as their aunt intervenes.

"Michael, you have been very strong throughout their lives, now is not the time to weaken."

"I know but these are my children you both must understand that…"

The emergency crew bring in three stretchers.

"What is happening?"

"Sir, we are going to take your children to the hospital." As they take each child, Michael shouts.

"Wait! I must call their doctors!"

"Sir, they have been notified. It is imperative that we leave immediately."

"Okay, Yolanda I'm going with… Oh God, I can't decide!"

"Michael, go with Annabelle; Aunt Ruthie and I will meet you at the hospital."

"Okay Yolanda."

As Michael looks at each of his children, he rushes to Annabelle's side. As he goes outside, he sees three ambulances there waiting to take his children away, and then panic starts to set in.

"Oh, my Lord, no!"

"Sir, please keep moving. We must leave."

As onlookers stand on the street to see what is happening, they watch each child is being taken out on a stretcher. They all look in disbelief as they clasp their hands to their mouths, and Michael realizes that his biggest fear, his worst nightmare, is unfolding right before his very eyes but has no time to think as he jumps in the ambulance with Annabelle. The doors close, and they leave with the sirens blaring. He sits there, staring at Annabelle in the stretcher with IVs in her and an oxygen mask, and thinks about all his children in their ambulances looking the same, and he could do only one thing—pray.

"Father, Lord please help my children. Be by their sides as each one fights. Please be with them and help them. Father, although it is Sunday, you said at midnight, please I beg of you to not to take them now. I will do it, Father. I will do what is asked of me. Just please Father, help them. Please."

After what seemed like an eternity to Michael, they arrive at the hospital. The doors open, and as Michael jumps out, he sees that all three ambulances are there. One by one each child is taken into the hospital on stretchers as doctors and nurses are all there scrambling to each child. They speak Michael, and he tries to listen but cannot make out a single word. As he runs with his children, they each go back into the trauma unit, and he is stopped at the door by the staff.

"Sir we can't allow you to go through."

Michael heard what they had just said but couldn't comprehend the words coming out of their mouths. As he looks through the window, he sees each of his children being taking back farther and farther. He drops to his knees and tries to understand what has just transpired. Hours go by, and Michael continues to ask the staff about his children, and still no word. With the sun out blaring its rays, Michael looks out the door and realizes how quickly time is passing and that there is nothing he could do from there; he then goes out to the waiting room where he finds Yolanda and Aunt Ruthie.

"Michael, where are the children?"

"I don't know, Aunt Ruthie. When they were brought in, they were taken into the trauma unit, and the staff wouldn't let me in."

"What?" his aunt and sister both said. "Are they at least giving you updates?"

"No Aunt Ruthie. They don't know a thing yet."

"That's outrageous!" Yolanda screamed as she walks to the nurse's desk. "Excuse me! Who in their right minds keeps a father away from their children like this?! Who do you all think you are not to give my brother updates about his children?!"

"Ma'am, as I said to Michael, when we know something, we will give him an update. Please calm down."

"Excuse me?!"

"Yolanda, it's okay, they are doing their best they can do for them."

"That's unacceptable that they won't at least give you an update, Michael!"

"Yolanda, yelling at them will not change the fact that we are here. It's not their fault."

"Fine Michael."

"Ma'am, as I told Michael there is a family waiting room available. You all can wait in there, and when we get information someone will be in there to notify you as soon as possible."

"Thank you, nurse. Let's go in here and wait."

They go into the room and wait. Many more hours pass by, and Michael knew there was only one place that he needed to be other than with his children.

"Aunt Ruthie, Yolanda, there is somewhere I must be at now."

"No Michael. Wherever you are than so are we," Yolanda said sternly.

"I appreciate that, but please wait here with Aunt Ruthie so when there is an update you both will be here."

"Where are you going Michael?"

"Aunt Ruthie, the only place that makes any sense… church."

"Okay Michael. If you must go, then do so."

"Thank you."

"Michael, I will call you if their doctors come."

"They should call me regardless, but I appreciate that. I will see you guys soon."

Michael then walks back to the nurse's desk.

"Excuse me miss? Is there a chaplain that I can speak with?"

"There is, but he is on call. I can page him if you would like me to."

"No, that's okay. Is there a chapel around?"

"Yes, it's on the other side of the hospital. Just follow the signs. You can't miss it."

"Okay thank you."

Michael then makes his way to the chapel. As he walks through the hospital, he sees bed after bed passing him. Patient after patient. Doctor after doctor. He finally arrives and enters to find a lonely, deserted chapel. He then walks in, goes to the front and drops to his knees. No prayer, no tone, just silence. He looks up and sees decorative art in beautiful bronze. Jesus on the cross. As he stares at it, he starts to wonder what was going through Jesus's mind when he knew he had to bear the cross. As he sat there for a while thinking about that, he then hears the doors open and an elder chaplain wearing a black robe with a white satin tassel and two embroidered crosses enters.

"Oh, I apologize. Am I interrupting?"

"No father, please come in. I need to speak with someone. I'm lost now."

The chaplain walks in.

"We are all lost at some point, son. It's those that seek guidance are the ones that finds their way."

"I'm afraid not in this instance."

"Please have a seat." Michael sits with him. "What's troubling you?"

"Father, my children are here at the hospital fighting for their lives, and yet all I could think of doing was coming here to this chapel. What kind of father am I to do so?"

The chaplain smiles.

"A loving father."

"How can that be true? I should be close to them. Screaming and fighting with the staff on any and everything I can about my children, but for some reason, I felt a strong need to be in here. What kind of man would do that?"

"One who is strong in faith. Hospitals has a way of turning many people into the direction of where they can find faith."

"I have faith, father. I believe in our Father, and I have accepted Jesus Christ as my Lord and Savior."

"Shall we ask for guidance?"

"I know that our Father has a plan for us all. In fact, I have prayed, and my prayers have been answered, but the result is that for my family to feel happiness they must first endure pain."

"It sounds like you have some inside information that this book of mine isn't telling me."

"It's not that. It's just I know what the task is asked for me to do so."

"Somethings are only to our Father's will."

"I heard that many times the other night, but I am struggling with my faith on it."

"Then pray. Sometimes all our father wants from you is to remain faithful that he knows what he is doing. You see everything that happens in this world isn't an accident or a miracle but by God's design."

"I tell my children that all the time, but now I am very confused."

"Our Father puts us in situations and paths to show us that He is watching over us. Not to control us but to show us how loving He is."

"If that's the case, then why make us suffer? Why must we go through so much anguish? Why are my children fighting for their lives? I just don't understand it."

"Son, there isn't a quote or words that I can give you to make you think otherwise, but this good book in my hand is the best playbook that you can ever have. Trust me, it has helped me many times throughout my life. The words written in it have all the answers that you seek."

"Forgive me, father, but it may be a playbook for you but not for this situation. It's not written anywhere in it that explains away why three faithful, loving children are dying. Why a God-loving man must witness that? There are no answers written in there to what I seek."

"You must realize something. You are here in this chapel speaking with me instead of not only driving the staff but yourself crazy. Isn't that something?"

"Father, I know what you are trying to do, but I feel why test us? Why does God put us in such predicaments that we will feel anger toward him and not trust the fact that He knows what He is doing?"

"Faith will set you free from everything that you do not understand. Trust in our Father, and the answers that you seek will follow. Unfortunately, there are too many times that I have questioned our Father, but I prayed on it. I know that I am not perfect, and He understands that because our Father is a perfect, loving God and whenever I am lost, He will wait for me to find Him again."

"You, father?"

"Yes, do you think I was born a minister with a bible clutched in my hands? No, but He waited for me. Doesn't that sound like a loving God?"

"Yes, but father you are here now. At least you have the privilege of knowing your fate. I on the hand along with my children are not too sure about."

"That's the thing—although you may not be sure, our Father is, and He will always be understanding. He will wait for you. Trust and believe in His plan, because He trusts and believes in you."

"Thank you father, and I am sorry if I sounded like I wasn't understanding you."

"It was my pleasure speaking with you, and whatever task our Father is asking of you, know that He would never give it to you unless He knew that you can handle it."

Michael thinks back to the conversation with the angel and notices the similarities in that which he just spoke with the chaplain. With a confused look, he softly says, "Angel?"

The chaplain smiles.

"No, my son. I am just a man in this chapel seeking guidance as well. Maybe it came in the form of speaking with you."

"Thank you, father."

"Peace be with you. I will say a prayer for you and your family. May God bless you."

"Thank you, father."

As the chaplain left the chapel, Michael knew in fact what must happen to heal his children and what must become of it. He then looks at the cross again, but this time he understood what Jesus must have been thinking when he was given the task of bearing the cross.

"Lord forgive me for what I must do."

Nighttime has now come, and hours had passed since Michael had left his sister and aunt. Still dazed on what he must do to save his children, he can only think of all the memories he has with them but also their illnesses. He then gets a call.

"Hello?"

"Michael, it's Yolanda. Where are you? Doctor Smith is here, and he needs to speak with you."

"I'm sorry. Please tell him that I am on my way."

"Hurry Michael."

"I'm coming."

Michael can only think of the worst, as any parent would. He makes his way to them and as he does, he gets another call.

"Hello?"

"Hello. Michael?"

"Yes…"

"It's Doctor Lee. I need to speak with you immediately."

"Okay I am almost there. I am coming to see Doctor Smith, as well. Wait there I'm coming."

Michael then rushes to them all while his mind starts to race, and he tries to rationalize the situation.

"Okay that must be a good sign that two doctors want to speak with me, right?" Then his mind wanders. "But what about Doctor Gomez? She hasn't called. How is Annabelle? Why hasn't her doctor called yet?"

After what seems like an eternity for him to get there, he arrives to find a frantic Yolanda who comes up to him.

"Michael, where were you?!"

"I just needed to get away and have a conversation with God, but I am here now. What's going on with my children?""

"I don't know, they wouldn't tell us anything. All they could say is that they needed to speak with you first. Michael, go find out what is going on!"

"Okay, I'm on it."

As Michael walks, he holds his breath on what he might hear. He goes up to the first of his children's doctors that he sees.

"Doctor Smith, how is Gabriel? Is he okay? Please tell me something. What's wrong with him?"

"Michael, I need you to have a seat."

"No, doctor. Just please tell me."

"Gabriel is stable. I gave him pain medicines and some medicines to help him get comfortable."

"Comfortable? For what?!"

"As I said to you when you were in my office, by the time he was diagnosed with DSRCT, his tumor had already spread to his other organs, and they are failing."

"What?!"

"Michael, I already discussed with you that someone with DSRCT only has a 15 percent, five-year survival rate."

"He just got diagnosed doctor! That means he has at least has five years!"

"Michael, his condition is so rare that there isn't enough definitive information to go on. Research on it has only gotten so far. His treatments were helping him cope at best. I'm sorry, Michael, I don't expect Gabriel to survive for very long."

Michael stood there in shock and couldn't come up with words. He tried to grasp what the doctor had just told him.

"I will remain here, making sure that he is comfortable and suffers minimal pain during his time here. I'm afraid that is the only comfort that I can provide for you now. I'm truly sorry Michael."

As the doctor walks away, Michael stood there speechless and fought every urge to panic. Yolanda and Aunt Ruthie came up to him.

"Doctor where are you going? Michael, what is going on with Gabriel?"

All he could do is cry.

"Michael, what is it?"

"Yolanda, Aunt Ruthie, the doctor doesn't expect Gabriel to live long."

"Oh my Lord… no." As they tear up, they run to the doctor and plead for him to examine Gabriel again, and it was then that Michael realized he still must speak with Jazmyn's doctor. He goes up to her and speaks softly.

"Doctor Lee… what's going on with my Jazmyn? Is she okay?"

"Michael, after looking over her charts and taking account from her illness, it is my medical opinion that Jazmyn will need a kidney."

"A what?!"

"You must understand, Michael, that her cancer is not only rare but an aggressive one. That is the reason why she was unresponsive. I have already submitted the paperwork but to be frank, there are many children that need a kidney and, given her age, it will not be easy."

"She is only three! That must account for something!"

"It does, but children with this illness above 18 months suffer from long-term effects if they survive. If she is able to get a kidney, then it's more like a blessing in disguise."

"So, it's either maybe she will get this kidney, or if not then she will suffer long-term effects?! Is that what you are telling me?!"

"Yes, Michael. I wish I could give you hope, but I am someone with medical facts, and the facts are if Jazmyn doesn't get one then it's not going to be good. Just put it in God's hands."

"May I see her?"

"Yes, she is heavily medicated, but you may see her."

"Thank you, doctor. Can you please tell my sister and aunt?"

"Of course, Michael."

He just stood there trying hard not to react as he watches his sister and aunt in shock over what the doctor is telling them. He knew there was one doctor left to see…Doctor Gomez. He then goes to the nurse's desk sobbing.

"Excuse me nurse? Can you please tell me if there is any word on my daughter Annabelle?"

"I will take a look."

"Thank you."

As she looks on the computer, he stood there in tears.

"I'm sorry Michael but you must speak with her doctor. She will be out shortly."

"What?"

"I can't say any more than that, I'm sorry."

"Okay, thank you."

His sister and aunt come to him in tears.

"Look guys, I know that what you both are hearing is tough, but I need you both now more than anything. I'm going to see Jazmyn and then going to see Gabriel."

"Of course, Michael."

"We are here for you Michael."

"Thank you both and also if…" Michael looks over and sees Doctor Gomez and immediately runs to her. "How is my Annabelle?"

"Michael we must speak in private." She looks to the nurse. "Can you find us somewhere secluded that we may have a quiet place to speak?"

"Right away, doctor."

Michael cannot hold his emotions.

"No! I heard enough about my children's futures slimming!"

"Michael, we must speak in private."

"No doctor! Just tell me what all of you already know!"

"Michael, Annabelle is in a medically induced coma."

"What?! What do you mean medically induced?!"

"Annabelle is far too unstable, so I made the executive decision to put her under."

"Who gave you the right?! Who told you that you can do that?! I certainly didn't authorize that! Now my daughter is in a coma! Did you at least consult with the other doctors on it?! Unless…" Michael realizes the situation and sobs. "That was your only option."

"Michael, I understand what you must be feeling now."

"No doctor, you don't."

"You must understand by doing so it was the only way of saving her life. I exhausted all other options before I made the decision to put her under. I gave her everything she needs to feel…"

Michael interrupts.

"Please do not say comfortable doctor!"

"Michael, this was our only option for saving your daughter. Please understand in situations like this, it was deemed necessary."

"What do you mean situations?!"

"Michael, I am sorry to say this, but she wasn't expected to live this long. Annabelle is in danger of having a heart attack and God only knows what else."

"You're right about one thing doctor! God does know! Not you! Not all these people! Not this hospital! Only God does!"

"Michael, I had already told you to cherish your time with her well. I'm afraid we are at the end."

"With all your specialty and years of practicing medicine, out of all the medical staff here, and out of all the medicine here at this hospital at your disposal. You are standing there and telling me that this is the end?!"

"I am afraid so Michael. Go spend what may be in fact your last moments with your daughter. I am sorry Michael."

Michael stood there and felt a rage that he never experienced before, but before he could act on it, he knew exactly what must be done to save his children. The task that was asked of him from our Father. He gathered all three doctors together with tears falling down his cheeks and asked them all one of the most difficult questions to ask, one that he didn't want to hear the answer to.

"Doctors, I know all of you spoke amongst each other about my children. I want to know, in your medical opinions, who in your eyes will not make it come Monday morning."

As the doctors looked at each other, Michael watched their faces immediately turn to sorrow as they one by one said the name that Michael knew it would be all along.

"Annabelle."

"Annabelle."

"I'm sorry Michael, it's Annabelle."

Michael, being the strong, faithful man that he is couldn't take what they just said and just cried out loud.

"No! Not my sweet innocent Annabelle!" He continued softly. "Please God… not her." Michael pleaded and begged the doctors, but they already came to that conclusion some time ago—Annabelle wasn't going to survive. Michael dropped to his knees, knowing that it was Annabelle who God wanted to return home all along, and he can only summon enough strength to ask her doctor one more question.

"Can I see my daughter, doctor?"

"Of course, Michael, but understand that she may not be able to respond to you. I'm sorry Michael."

He picks himself up and runs to her room. He just stands there crying and staring at his daughter, Annabelle.

"I'm so sorry this is happening to you sweetie. I love you so much, and I know that your brother and sister love you just as much. I must go see them sweetie. You just keep dreaming. Please don't go anywhere. I will be back sweetie." Michael kisses her on her forehead, then he looks in disbelief at what is happening to her. He looks at the clock on the wall and realizes that midnight is fast approaching.

"I will be back to say goodbye."

He then goes to his princess where he finds a groggy, heavily medicated Jazmyn laying in her bed.

"Daddy…"

"Hey princess, you're awake. How are you feeling?"

"Sickie Daddy… sickie."

"I know princess, but guess what? The doctors said you are going to be okay."

"Promise…"

"I promise princess. Did you have fun at the park yesterday?"

"Yeah."

"Remember all the animals we were able to see? Remember Cartoon Land? I want you to remember all the fun we had together as a family. I will also promise you that next time you go you will be able to ride the rides."

She begins to close her eyes.

"Yay… tired Daddy…tired."

"It's all going to be okay princess. You rest your beautiful eyes and go to dream land."

As she falls asleep, Michael stares at her thinking of everything that she will become, all the experiences, all the memories. He kisses her on the forehead and whispers, "I love you so much princess. Rest up for tomorrow. You will be healed. These doctors don't know a thing, because I only answer to a higher authority. I love you."

As he leaves, he looks back one more time and wipes his tears away. He then is meet by a sobbing aunt at the door.

"Hey, Aunt Ruthie, please remain here so when she wakes, she is not alone."

"Of course, Michael. I'm not going anywhere."

"Thank you for everything that you have done for us. You know, I think she loved you more than Yolanda and me," he joked with tears in his eyes.

"Michael, don't say that. She loves all of us just the same," she said, wiping her tears.

"It's okay, Aunt Ruthie. I wouldn't have it any other way."

As she walks in to sit with Jazmyn, Michael gathers himself and prepares to go see his son. He then goes to his room and opens the door. Not knowing what to expect, he see a heavily medicated Gabriel laying in his bed.

"Daddy... you came."

"Of course I did buddy. Where else would I rather be but here with you?"

"Daddy, I feel funny."

"It's okay buddy, the doctors gave you some magic potion to make the meanies go away."

"Did we kick their butts, Daddy?"

"You sure did buddy, but there are still more butts to kick."

"Okay."

"Buddy, you are a soldier, so I need you to fight and be so strong that the meanies won't know when you kick their butts."

"Yeah, Daddy. I'm going to win, right?"

"You sure are buddy, and I promise you that when you wake up tomorrow morning that you won't even remember what it felt like to have meanies."

"Promise, Daddy?"

"I promise buddy, but I need you to fight with all your might right now."

"Okay, Daddy, anything for you, but the meanies are hurting me right now. Can you tell the meanies to leave me alone?"

"You meanies better leave my little buddy alone. Better buddy?"

"It hurts Daddy."

Michael presses the help button.

"I just called in someone to help you beat up the meanies. I need you to fight buddy."

"Okay Daddy… okay." In comes the nurse.

"Did you call?"

"Yes, my little buddy is in pain. Can you please help him?"

"Of course. It's actually time for his medicine. I was on my way here to give it to him when I saw the light on outside his room."

"Sorry about that."

"No, it's okay. Hey little guy. Are you hurting?"

"Yeah."

"Okay I have something here that will help you." She injects the medicine into his I.V.

"There you go little guy. That should make it feel all better and sleepy too. So that you can sleep good tonight."

"Thank you."

"You're welcome. Is there anything else that you need?"

"No."

"Okay little guy. You get some rest."

"Thank you, nurse."

"No problem. He should be asleep here in a few minutes. I will be coming in and out throughout the night, keeping an eye on him. If there is anything else that you need just press the call light."

"Okay, thank you."

She then leaves, and Michael just looks at Gabriel as he goes in and out, fighting his sleep.

"Hey buddy. I know that I told you to fight and be strong, but if you need to sleep then rest. I only want you to fight for me by not going anywhere but off into dreamland."

"Okay Daddy. I'm here. I'm your little buddy."

Michael's voice breaks and tears fill his eyes. He can only softly speak.

"You sure are buddy… you sure are."

Gabriel closes his eyes and falls asleep. Michael just stares at his son, thinking of all the wonderful things that will happen for him, every laughter that he will get to experience from being cancer free. He then kisses him on his forehead and, with tears in his eyes, he walks out the room to find a teary-eyed Yolanda standing there.

"Hey sis, please do me a favor and stay with my little buddy. The nurse will be in and out throughout the night, but if he needs anything or wakes in pain, then hit the nurse light and she will come."

"Anything, Michael. If he needs anything at all I will call someone in, and if they don't then may God have mercy on their souls." Michael smiles with tears in his eyes.

"I believe you will, sis. Thank you for everything that you do for us. We couldn't be a family without you. I just wanted you to know that. There is something that I must do, so I will be with Annabelle in her room. I love you sis."

"I love you too, Michael. Go do whatever you must do. Go be with her."

"Thank you, Yolanda."

She walks into Gabriel's room and sits down with him. Michael then goes to the one room that he knew he must be in—Annabelle's. As he walks in, he just stares at her, even though there were machines everywhere making all the sounds, he looked at her laying there looking like she was sleeping peacefully. Feeling no pain, no sickness. He then wonders if that is what it's like in heaven and begins to speak with her in a soft tone with tears in his eyes.

"Sweetie, I know that you are more than likely talking to Jesus now, but I need for you to hear me. I am sorry for all the pain that you have gone through. I am sorry for the fact that I couldn't take this illness away from you myself, because if I were able to, I would have. Will you remember me sweetie? Will you remember your family? I know now why God wants you back home, because you are an angel walking amongst us humans. This world wasn't ready for your beauty, laughter, your soul. Your laughter alone was so contagious that it was an amazing thing to hear." He begins to cry. "And I am so sorry that I won't be able to hear it again. Sweetie, I am going to miss you so much. I am going to miss not being able to like any of your boyfriends, because I know nobody out there is good enough for you.

I am going to miss watching you looking ever so beautiful in your dress walking down the aisle. Sweetie, I am so sorry." Michael begins to cry uncontrollably. "I do know that you will never feel the pain from your illness anymore. Please don't ever forget about us. I want you to always remember how much I love you, okay? Please don't ever forget that. Always remember that you have my heart from the day you were born when I first held you. Of course, you had to share it with your brother and sister, but I want you to remember that. Please be careful with it and no matter where you are, I want you to sing like you never sang before and dance like you never danced before. Sweetie, never stop knowing how deeply you are loved both here on earth and in heaven. I love you, Annabelle."

As he sat there in silence crying, he felt a warmth touch on his shoulder and knew exactly who it was.

"Is she with our Father yet?" he asked softly. "Is she walking with Jesus?"

Michael turns to the angel with tears in his eyes.

"No, Michael, she hasn't left yet but soon she will never know the pain from her illness. None of your children will as promised to you from our Father. Soon she will leave this world and once again you all will be reunited."

"When she leaves will she feel anything?"

"Just the gentle hand of Jesus as he walks her home and the love of all those waiting for her in the kingdom of heaven."

"Will she remember us?"

"Michael, God has blessed all of you here on Earth as equals to have one another. As brothers and sisters. As you all share that here in this world, we do as well in the kingdom. So, if you are asking me if she will remember you as her father then yes Michael, she will, and when she sees you, she will run up to you with open arms. Michael, you and your family were created to be just that—a family—and you all will be such as much in the kingdom of heaven when you all are reunited with each other."

"Anna as well?"

"Yes Michael, all of you will be reunited. Everything you have on Earth—the love, laughter, happiness—is in heaven. All you living beings will be together."

"Animals?"

"Even animals, Michael. You think they are without souls? Anything that is created by God here on Earth is in heaven. Add that to the list of wonderful, amazing, creations that I cannot explain to you. All of it, Michael, is waiting on you in heaven."

"So, is it true about what animal Jesus has?"

"His horse? Yes Michael, it's so beautiful and majestic that I am not allowed to tell you more about it unless he shows his beautiful animal to you. I know with the love that Annabelle has for all beings she will love the kingdom and all of its beauty."

"I know that she will love it there. May I ask you something?"

"Sure."

"I know we call him our Father, but is God a he or she? There is a lot of debate here on Earth about that subject."

"That's the problem. Most that do not understand a higher power try to analyze and label something that they do not understand. God is neither a he nor she. Our father is a divine power of love radiating throughout this world and above. Just look at your children. Isn't that proof enough?"

Michael looks at Annabelle.

"Yes, they are proof of God's love. May I ask you another question?"

"Anything."

"Did Anna know?"

"That she was going home? If I tell you yes, will that change anything?"

"No, you're right about that, but one thing has been troubling me about her departure."

"Only one?"

"Did she know about everything and is that why she secretly took out an insurance policy on herself—because she knew I would be here with our children to take care of them?"

"Michael, you know the answer to your question."

Michael looks at Annabelle.

"Yes, she knew. Anna always knew what was best for her family. Please don't allow Annabelle to forget me."

"She never will. You are her father. You showed her and all your family a love that only our Father shows. Michael, I am sorry, but it is midnight, and I must obey our Father by His ruling. It has been written, Michael. Our Father knows of your decision, but I need to make sure that you are ready to live by this decision. Do not fear, for Annabelle will be at peace once again. All your children will, as promised. It's time Michael. Are you ready for your decision?"

"I am. I love you sweetie. Please keep me in your memory."

A bright light appears and engulfs the room. The angel walks with the one who Michael had decided on, and as they walk into the light a voice speaks.

"Welcome, my child. I have been waiting for you."

As fast as the light appeared, it vanished. All that remained in the room was one lifeless body and one full of life. The medical team rushed in, but they were too late. The soul is already in the presence of our Father.

Three days have passed, and Michael is standing in a church filled with mourners, admiring how beautiful it is as he looks at all the photos that are placed in the entry way. He sees the coffin, which he did not want to see but knew he must. He begins to walk slowly down the aisle, his shoes echoing throughout the church. As he gets closer to the coffin, he takes in of all those that have attended. He sees his brother and cousins, dressed in their dress blues.

"Guys, do not look so sad. Although this may feel like a tragedy, we must celebrate the miracle that came from this." The only response he receives from them is sadness. Michael then walks to the front row to see his aunt sitting there quietly as she tries to wipe her tears away.

"Aunt Ruthie, help me out. Please tell them to stop mourning and celebrate the miracle." She puts her head down and begins to feel the pain of losing someone she saw as one of her own. He then turns to his sister.

"Yolanda, I do not understand? I know it's painful right now, but everyone here should be celebrating the lives saved, not mourning a life lost, because it's not. This is not the end of a life but the beginning of a new one. You, of all people, should know where I am coming from, right sis?"

All she could do is stare at the coffin and cry. Michael sees what she is looking at, slowly walks up to the coffin, and looks inside with hesitation to see what he did not want to see… a lifeless body lying there. He realized that without a soul, it was just a vessel. All he could do was admire how peaceful it looked and comment on how beautiful a job they did with it. He then turned around to see his children sitting there in pain and he tried to comfort them.

"Shh princess, please do not cry. Look! No more bubble, no more sickie. You will grow up to be the queen you are meant to be and rule this world one day, but remember you will always be daddy's little princess. Okay?"

Overcome with pain, she could only cry. He then goes to Gabriel.

"Buddy, I know that you are sad now, but trust me it will get better. Look at you, my big strong soldier who beat up the meanies. You did it buddy! No more meanies as promised. No more doctors, no more magic lasers. Now you can race big cars all you want! I know that you may not comprehend this now, but remember what I had said about it feeling like sometimes it seems like it's going to rain forever? Always remember the sun will come out again and shine ever so brightly for you. Okay?"

Gabriel, feeling the pain of losing someone he loves dearly, just sits there and cries out. Michael, feeling their pain as well, turns to the casket once more and then kneels in front of Annabelle as she sits there next to her brother and sister, feeling the sorrow of losing their father and crying along with them.

"Sweetie, I know that you are going through so many emotions right now, but I need you to know that this is how much I love you all. I said this to you all many times, but love really is the most powerful weapon on this earth. Although this doesn't make sense now, you all must understand the only way to prove my love is by sacrificing myself for you guys. You probably will not understand this now, but you will realize one day that I did this so that you guys will not have to go to adventure land anymore. No more magic potions, no more medicines. You, your brother, and your sister can all live freely now without worrying about these illnesses because they are gone. Isn't that something sweetie?!" Michael's tears begin to fall. "

I need you to look after your brother and sister from now on. I trust and believe in you, Annabelle. I always have. Remember all that I have taught you and never forget family is the most important thing to have in this world. I know your ears can't hear what I am saying to you right now, but I know your hearts can. So please understand when I say this: I will always be there for you soldiers. Whenever you need me, I will be there for you all. Stay strong and keep your aunts on their toes for me." Michael smiles as he wipes his tears. "I love you sweetie." Suddenly a bright light appears, and Michael sees Anna standing there smiling.

"Anna my love, I missed you so much. I have been waiting for this moment ever since you left us."

"I never left, Michael. I have always been here with you all in your hearts just as you are never leaving. Yes, we will be home, but we will always be in their hearts and memories."

"I understand that and am happy to go home, but I just have so much guilt."

"Why do you have guilt?"

"For causing them this much pain, but this was the only way I could heal our children. I am terribly sorry they must endure this pain, but what's comforting is that they now have a clean slate. Our children can experience life as they were meant to—pain-free, illness-free. I keep justifying my decision by thinking any person given this opportunity would have done the exact same thing for their loved one."

"Only someone whose heart is filled with love, Michael. I knew that about you the first time I looked into your eyes. Our Father knew of your love the moment he created you." Michael smiles.

"I still do not understand something… Angel said God knew of my decision, but how can that be if I did not know until that very moment?" Anna smiles.

"Michael, our Father knew before you were born. He knew the way you looked at our children as you held them when they were born. Our Father knew the minute he gave you this task that this was the decision you were going to make. It was you, Michael, that God wanted to come home, not our children."

"Why me?"

"Your purpose in life was fulfilled."

"How was it fulfilled?"

"You taught our children not only about God but the power of His love and the strength it carries. You instilled faith, hope, and love into them, and they will carry those traits with them wherever they go in life. That, Michael, was your purpose in life. You were past your time here on Earth, but God loves you so much that He gave you extra time to be with our children." Michael and Anna both look at their children.

"They are so beautiful and perfect."

"They are indeed. Don't worry, Michael, we will all be together again in the kingdom of heaven one day."

"I love how that sounds."

Anna extends her hand to Michael.

"Are you ready to go home?"

Michael turns to look at their children one last time and smiles.

"I am."

Michael and Anna walk hand in hand into the light to go home.